Jenergy

THE ONLY WAY TO A FIT, FIRM AND FEMININE BODY

Jenergy

JENNI RIVETT

HarperCollins*Illustrated*

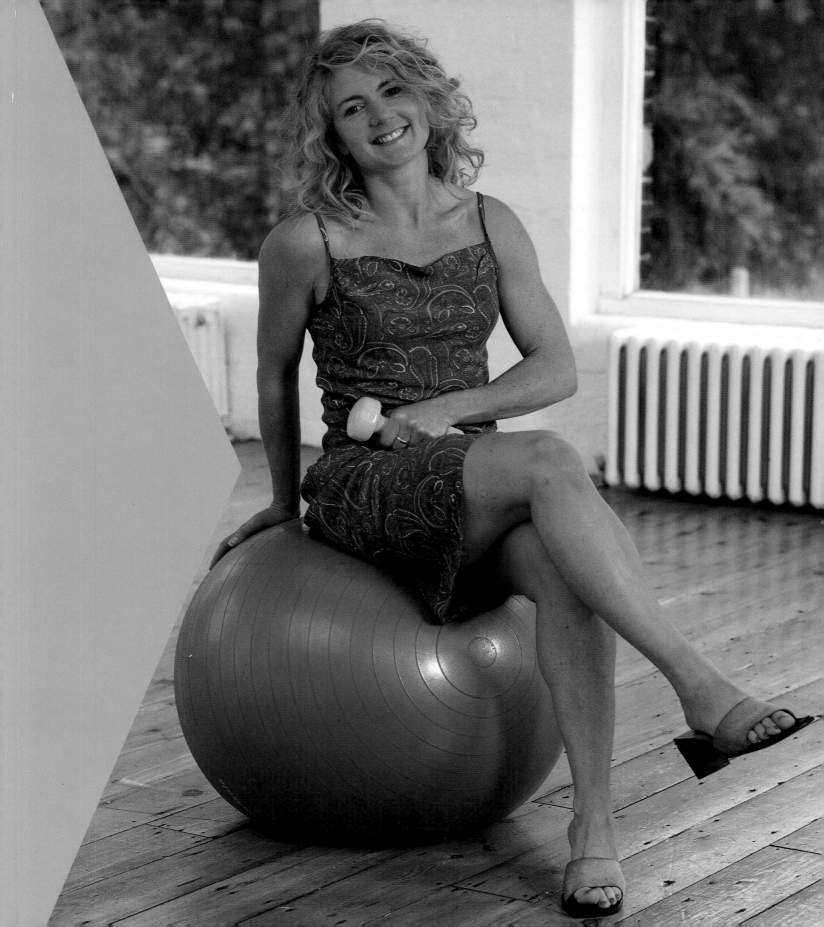

Contents

▶ ▶ ▶ ▶▌

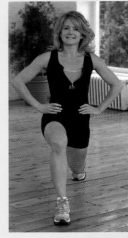

First Published by HarperCollins*Illustrated* 2001

An imprint of HarperCollins*Publishers*
77-85 Fulham Palace Road
London W6 8JB

The HarperCollins website address is
www.**fire**and**water**.com

Text © Jenni Rivett

Photographs © Guy Hearn

Design by Tanya Devonshire-Jones

ISBN: 0 00 711066 9

Colour origination by Colourscan, Singapore

Printed and Bound by Scotprint, Haddington.

Disclaimer

The authors of this book have made every effort to ensure
that the information contained in this book is as accurate and
as up-to-date as possible at the date of publication. However,
any information or advice should not be relied upon as
statements or representation of fact. The exercise programme in
this book is intended for people in good health, however, all
guidelines and warnings should be read carefully. If you have a
medical condition or are pregnant, the exercises in this book should
not be followed without first consulting a doctor. The author and
publisher cannot accept liability for any loss, damage or injury incurred as
a result (directly or indirectly) on the advice or information contained in this
book or the use or application of the contents of this book.

Foreword

By Lorraine Kelly

Thank goodness for the Jenergy programme! This has become part of my life. It is easy to maintain and more importantly, it works. I have to admit that I am not someone who loves to exercise, and I have never been able to stick to a diet. So I was sceptical when Jenni and I were asked to do a fitness video together. However, after grasping Jenni's philosophy it made more sense to me than anything else I have ever tried and I was therefore willing to give it a go. I have not looked back.

Yes, I go off track from time to time but Jenni has taught me how to get right back on the programme again without allowing it to turn into a downward spiral and it still amazes me that the weight does not pile on. I try really hard to eat sufficient amounts of healthy food throughout the week and relax a little more on the weekend. However, what I am finding is that the fitter and healthier I get, the less I want to eat junk food anyway. The exercise is the part that has probably made the biggest difference to me. After initially giving me one out of ten for technique, she now gives me ten out of ten. I now realise that this factor alone is what can really change your body shape. I power walk two or three times a week to keep my body fat down and knowing how to exercise properly makes it easy to fit a quick stomach or arm routine into my day.

I want every woman out there to know that this is a forever health and fitness routine that simply gets easier to sustain as your body gets fitter and your metabolism increases.

'Jenergy is the future of health and fitness.'

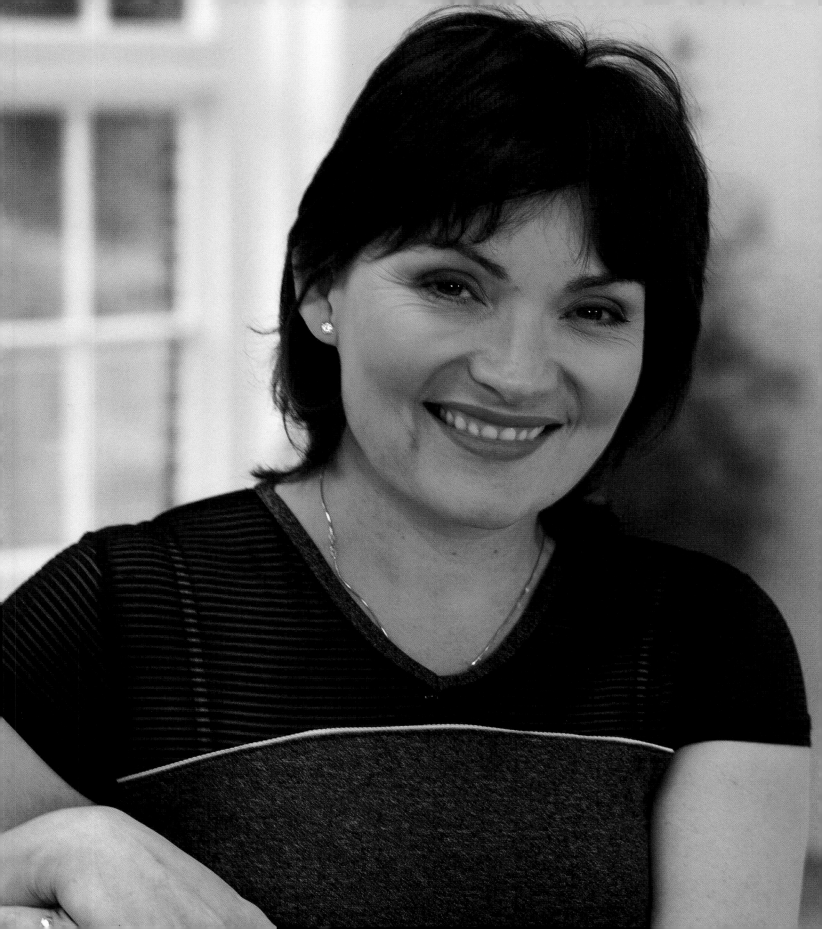

STOP

RIGHT THERE!

- *Fitness and health in the new century*

- *A personal trainer in your own home*

- *Achieve a fit, firm and feminine body*

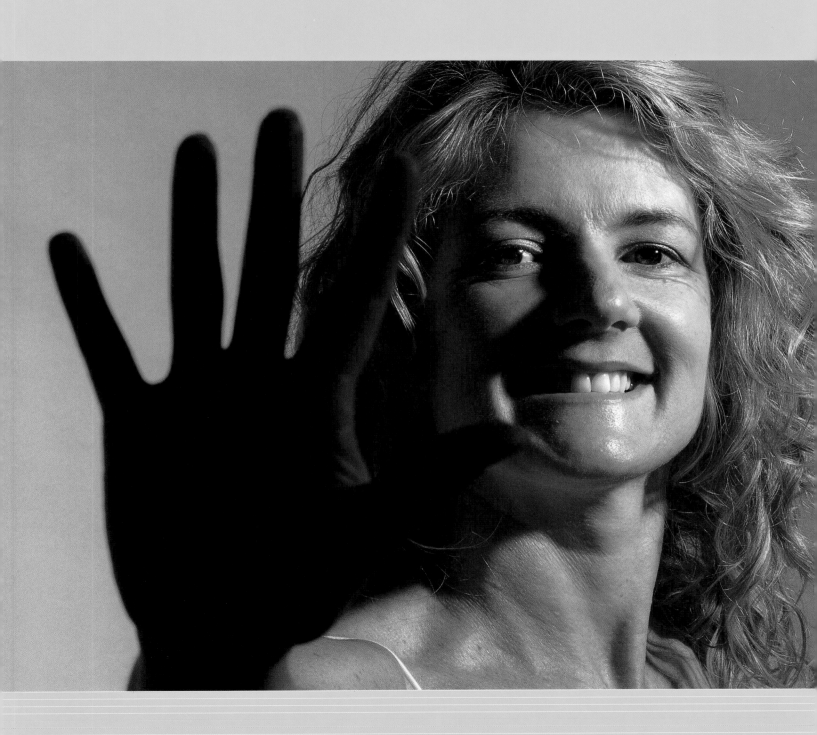

A New Body

So, here you are reading yet another book on how to achieve the body of your dreams. You are sitting on your favourite sofa, cup of coffee and three biscuits in one hand, whilst the other frantically searches the pages hoping to find a miracle weight-loss cure. Could there be some new tablet to dissolve fat whilst sitting on sofas devouring biscuits? Or perhaps it's been discovered that just five minutes of exercise a day will melt the pounds off. Or wait . . . what was that cabbage diet everyone was raving about? 'Whatever it is,' I sadly hear you say 'it's going to be hell'. 'After all, being permanently fit and slim is one of the most unattainable goals, isn't it?'

Why is it that women constantly look for the most difficult options to get fit and healthy? Perhaps you've been brainwashed into thinking only a 'gifted few' have great figures. They've inherited their genes. They come from an athletic background. They were born skinny. You have big bones. Your mother had a weight problem at your age. You've had four kids. You've had one kid. You have a thyroid problem. Your knees are dodgy so exercise is out of the question. The script goes on.

Are you on the never-ending roller coaster of diets? Have you given up on exercise because it doesn't seem to budge a pound? You start out with all good intentions and soon become disillusioned with lack of results. We have almost reached the stage where we want to be told we can only lose weight by stapling our stomach or having a 24-hour personal trainer – not surprising, when we look at the array of garbage hurled at us daily through the media and advertising. The dieting industry is worth billions of dollars and yet Americans and Britons are at their fattest ever. Stick-thin models adorn the covers of magazines making even a relatively fit, healthy person feel positively overweight. Every year some new expert proudly announces the latest gadget or diet. Enthusiastic yet vulnerable, you give into temptation only for your illusions to be shattered once again. They say women are 'shopaholics'. We might just as well be called 'dietaholics' too. Why do we continue to allow the dieting industry to convince us they have all the answers? Because *now* is appealing when we have three days to get into that slinky little black number. *Now* is what these fly-by-nights promise and in the end tears are what they deliver.

It is downright confusing to know exactly what to eat, which diet to follow, what exercise routine works best and so on. Everyone claims to have done the latest research on why carbohydrates make you fat or why not to eat meat and potatoes together. Just how long are you going to continue counting points or allowing yourself to tuck into some tasteless saccharine-pumped treat? How much longer are you going to hate what you see in the mirror and plan to start a diet next Monday? Do you really want to dread going to your husband's Christmas party year after year because your 500-a-day-calorie diet has failed yet again?

Women do constantly fail when it comes to their weight. Why? Two reasons: firstly, they try to be on a diet 100% of the time. When they don't succeed they allow it to turn into a week-long binge. Monday arrives and the cycle starts once again. You set yourself up for failure when you set goals that are extraordinarily high. Secondly, many women fail when it comes to exercise. This is because they either start out too vigorously and cannot sustain it, or they get bored. They get bored because they are not seeing results and they are not seeing results because they are exercising incorrectly.

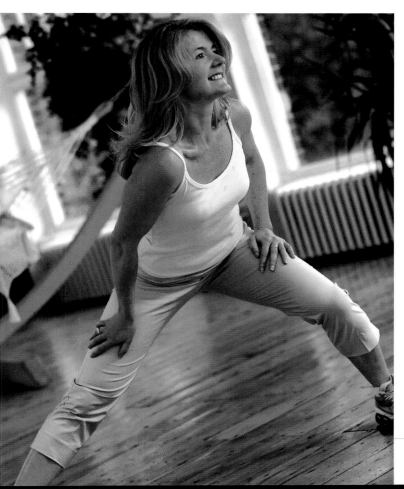

Yes, it certainly is going to take some convincing to get you to believe my system can and will get you in shape for life. After all, you've been let down once too often and have probably become quite sceptical about the real truth. I understand fully. An overweight teenager myself, I fast became an expert on the latest diet or exercise programme. Everything failed, and I eventually resorted to literally starving myself, living on little other than apples and tea. My health rapidly deteriorated and it took my descent to this very low point in my life to realise I was doing everything wrong.

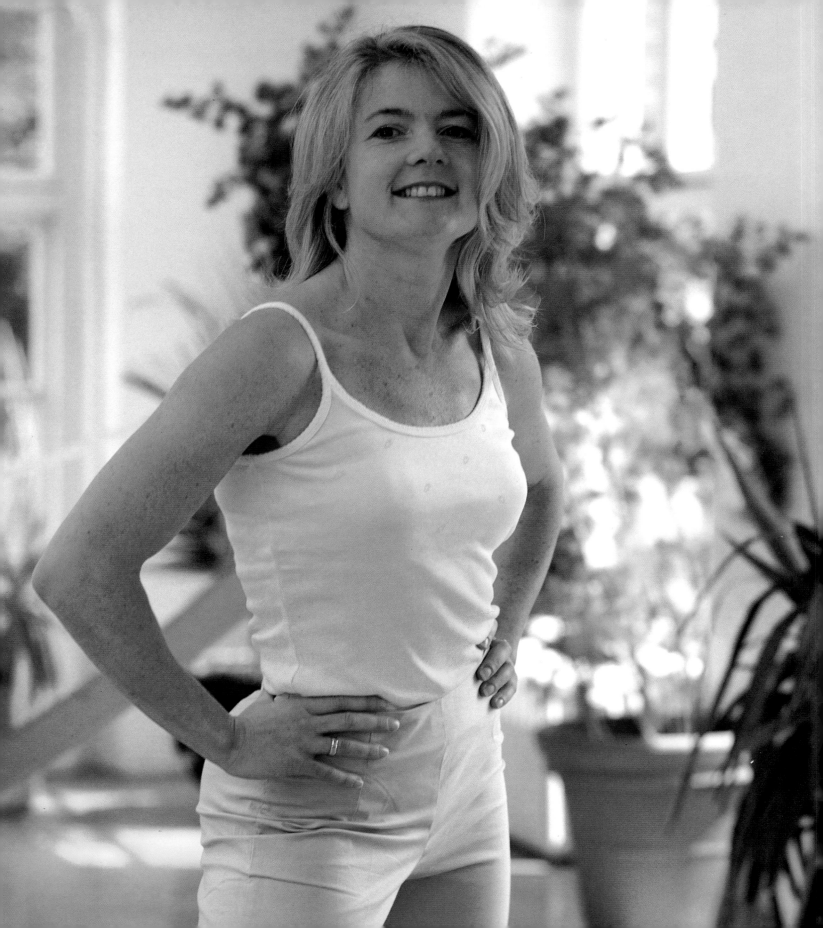

That was my turning point and now I feel fitter, healthier and more vibrant than I have ever felt. I am passionate about sharing my knowledge with you in the hope of helping you avoid the same painful path I endured for years. Armed with 15 years of experience and a huge success rate, my goal is to convince you that getting into shape is attainable. In addition, I will show you how to keep weight off forever. It's all a matter of understanding my principles and altering your previous pattern of thinking. My approach is simple and practical but, more importantly, it works. Once you educate yourself about the unique needs of your body and how it ticks, you will have acquired a most powerful tool which can become a reality in your life.

Using this book

This book is the closest I can get to being your personal trainer in your own home. Use it as your prescription for exercise and healthy eating. It's not about a seven-day diet. It's about re-educating yourself, changing your exercise plan, eating properly and then implementing it into your daily living. The major principles outlined in this book are where most women fail.

By really studying each principle carefully you will discover where and why you have failed in the past. Go through each section until you understand each and every concept. Correcting your exercise technique and getting off the dieting merry-go-round are the key factors to implementing permanent changes. You will understand that although important on their own, all the principles must link together to produce the final result which is a fit, firm, and feminine body that exudes super health and vitality.

'*My goal is to convince you that getting into shape is attainable.*'

The JENERGY WAY

- *Correct your technique*
- *Strength training*
- *A woman-only approach*
- *Maximise your fat blast*

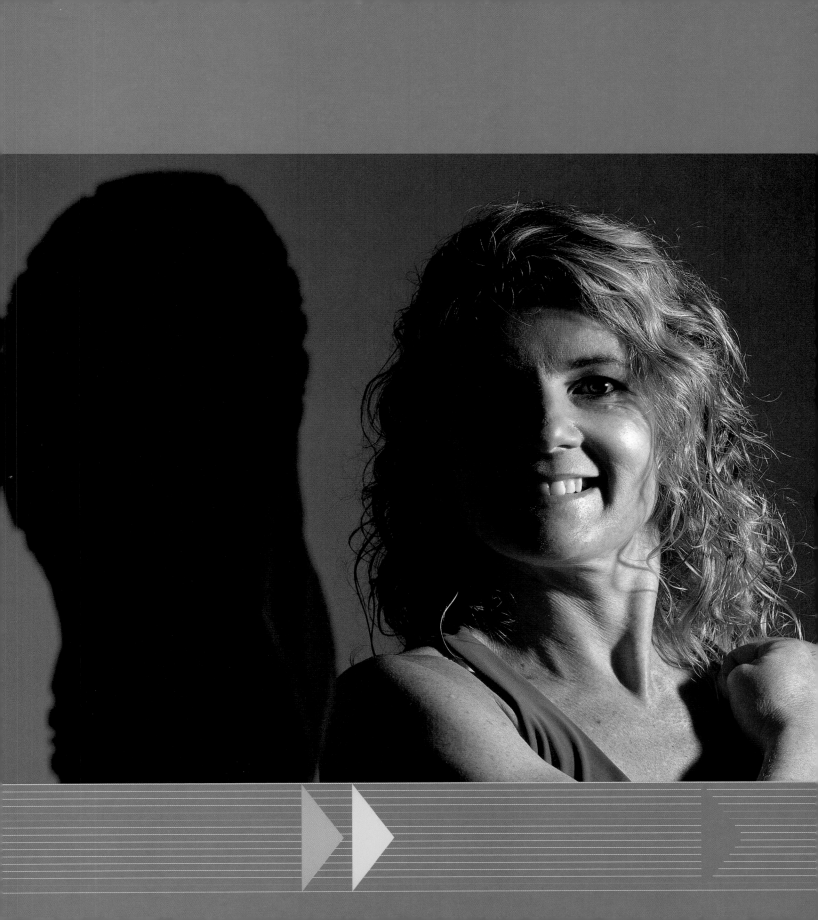

TECHNIQUE

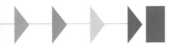

Technique is the number one factor in any fitness programme. You can wear the latest gear, work out on the highest of high-tech machinery, train regularly, but without perfect technique your body shape is unlikely to ever change, and you will become more susceptible to injury. In my experience, this is the area where most women fail.

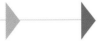

Douglas Brooks, world-renowned exercise physiologist and author of four major texts, agrees that the best resistance-training exercises should be chosen more for their 'correctness' than for their novelty. They should maximise effectiveness, safety, proper biomechanics, muscle function and client compliance.

Just recently, *New York* magazine said 'The culprits aren't the machines themselves – they're safe if used properly – but that they are used in laissez-faire gyms that are reluctant to tell amateurs they don't know what they're doing. Or that what they are doing – without the benefit of a $50-an-hour personal trainer, isn't going to give them the body they think they're getting.'

Correct your technique

Technique is very specific. It literally means moving a leg half an inch here or pushing your hips back more there. Simple as it is, this repositioning of the body makes all the difference to the end result. Like any new project or venture, you have to learn the technicalities before you can perfect it. For example, someone who has basic computer skills might take two hours to do something on the computer that a computer whiz could complete in half an hour. It is the same with your body. You could spend two years training, with minimal results, or seek the services of a professional and after two sessions, be well on the way to a great new body. Another very important factor relevant to technique is the actual quality of your movement whilst going through the motion. I put on a great comedy act imitating my class members during our monthly workshops. Showing them how *they* execute a move and how they *should* execute a move are two entirely different things. Every movement has to go through a certain range of motion and speed. If you move too quickly through a move, it will appear easy and you will also be stressing the joint rather than the muscle. This is the body's way of cheating by relying on the momentum rather than on controlling each move.

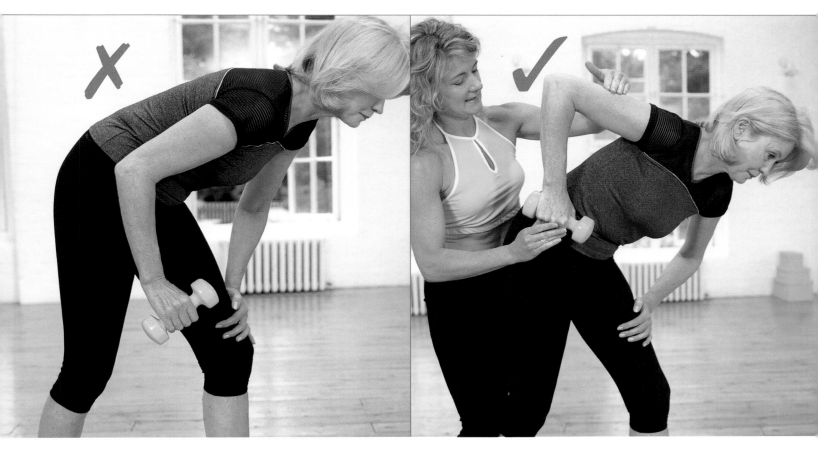

Poor posture, stance and incorrect arm positioning make this exercise totally ineffective.

Improving your posture and stance and correcting your arm position will produce the desired results.

Exercising incorrectly is like eating without tasting.

To prevent this from happening I encourage my clients to use the split-second technique. Every exercise has two movements, a start and a finish. Between the two movements hold the move for a split second and feel the muscle you are supposed to be working by squeezing it. Then control the movement on the way down. It's rather like making a fist and then squeezing your fist as hard as you can – you can literally feel the pressure building up.

Think about the martial arts guru Bruce Lee. He never worked out with weights. His beautifully sculpted body came just from working with his own body resistance. I often encourage my clients to try and work their muscles without weights so that they can really feel the muscles working by using their own strength and not relying on external strength. Try this basic exercise right now to understand this. Take your arm out to the side, up to shoulder level and down again. Simply swing it up and down several times. This is the way most people work their muscles. Now try this more controlled version. Lift your arm up to shoulder level, hold it there for a split second, squeezing through the shoulder and bring it back down with resistance. Do this several times and feel the difference. Now imagine implementing this technique into each and every exercise. Yep! A new body awaits you.

Repositioning of the body makes all the difference to the end result.

You have just learnt to correct your technique. By taking a muscle through a full range of motion you are working the full length of the muscle and will acquire the lean, lengthened look you desire. Working with short pulsing moves as in Callenetics prevents the muscles from being worked through a full range of motion.

Leave your thoughts of work or the kids behind. Without concentrating on the muscles you are supposed to be working you will not achieve the desired results. Each time you work a specific muscle focus your mind on doing the exercise correctly by feeling the muscle you are working.

By straightening your wrists, you will be working your biceps and not straining your forearms.

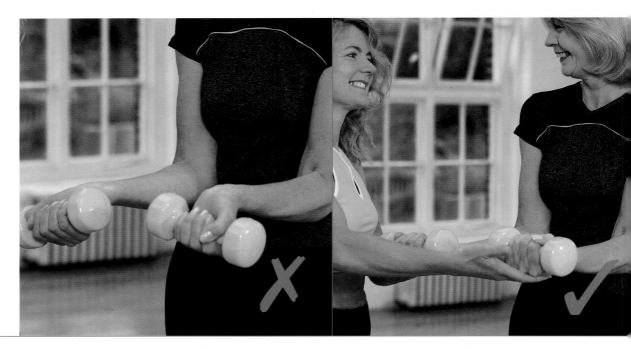

REAL WOMEN
and the Jenergy Way

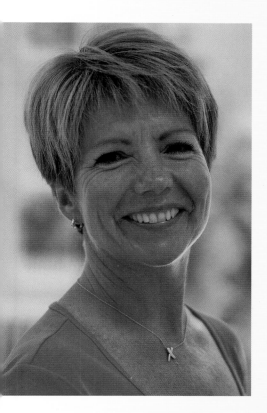

'I want to share this with the many women out there who are unable to change their body shape. It seemed impossible that I might be able to have a half way decent body let alone a great figure (which I now possess). And you know something, it was really easy. Yes, easy! All I did was change my technique and start exercising properly. It didn't quite evolve like that though. I had previously tried every new exercise class or fad so I was willing to give Jenni's class a try. After the third class, when I was just starting to lose interest, Jenni said something that altered my mindset forever. "If you don't think about the muscles you're working by concentrating on your technique, your body will be exactly the same in a year's time." What?

The intense realisation that the very thing I had avoided could be the key to a great body was a powerful motivator for me. After just three weeks of really concentrating on my technique with every exercise I started to notice the changes. I felt muscles I had never felt before. Jenni's technique proved I could achieve great results by exercising correctly, right in my own living room if I wanted. Ten months later, I'm a size 8. I've swapped my baggy sweaters for tight T-shirts and clothes shopping is fun again. Jenergy really works.'

WILMA KAUFMANN

Core stabilisation

Core stabilisation is all about creating strength through the central girdle: the abdominals, waistline, lower and middle-back muscles. When these muscles are weak and untoned posture is poor and it is very difficult to achieve the desired results whilst training other parts of the body. Call this mid-section of the body the chief and the other muscles the workers. If the chief is not sitting firmly on his throne demanding orders, his workers are going to slacken off. Similarly, if the central girdle is not in control whilst working other muscle groups, the results will be greatly reduced. Here's how to get in touch with working your central girdle correctly.

I view each part of the body separately to help me get muscles working both in tandem and on their own. The torso is my starting point. I teach clients to view this part of the body as a square. Straight across from the left shoulder to the right, down from the right shoulder to the bottom of the right hip (where the hip and thigh bone join), across to the left hip and back up to the left shoulder. This whole section of the body, both front and back, has a special and very focused task in each and every exercise performed.

The abdominal muscles are constantly held (not with force) towards the backbone. This creates torso stabilisation throughout all exercises and builds incredible strength through the abdominal and back muscles. Back-related pain costs companies millions of pounds every year as the number one reason for time taken off work. By implementing the principles underlined into your daily exercise and activity routines your back pain will become a thing of the past.

Core stablisation is all about keeping that square stationary whilst working the other body parts.

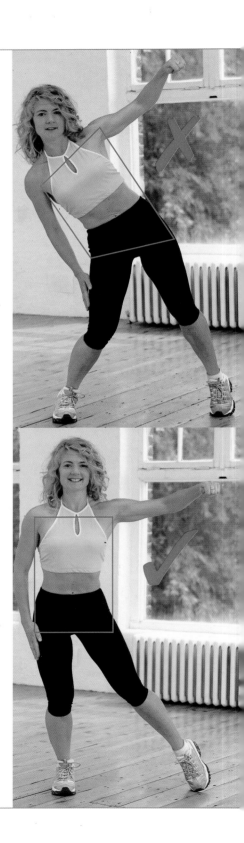

Once understood, the principles of core stabilisation will change the way you sit, stand, walk and work out in the future.

After grasping the concept of keeping the torso stable, I view the arms, legs and head as entirely separate from the square. The square constantly in place, we are now in a position to work all the other muscle groups with perfect technique. We take an arm and work an arm muscle without the interference of any other body part. We work the lower body with control, building perfect balance and strength through the legs. In other words, to gain the most benefit whilst working a specific muscle the square needs to be firmly in place. My favourite line to get this message across, and one you'll come across quite frequently in this book, is 'no other body part is invited to the party'. Stop jiggling the rest of your body around whilst you work a specific muscle. The only muscle moving is the one you are working. This does require a certain amount of practice and discipline but once mastered, it is never forgotten. This is an area where I see many women failing and is one of the first technicalities I correct. You will be amazed at the incredible control and power you have over your body once you learn core-stabilisation techniques. In addition, just by being aware of these muscles in everyday activities such as walking and standing will give you improved posture and make you look at least five pounds lighter.

Perfect posture and balance

Posture is normally described as neutral alignment – the ankles, knees, hips and shoulders are parallel to the floor, with a slight inward curve through the lower part of the spine and a slight outward curve in the thoracic level of the spine. Losing the ability to maintain neutral alignment during various activities causes most injuries. Sitting and standing incorrectly causes muscular imbalances in the body and affects posture and alignment.

Most of our balance skills are acquired at around the age of ten, but with poor muscle tone, coordination and posture we lose the intensity of our balance skills as we get older. This is true if you are out of shape. However, once you start to increase your muscle mass and gain control over your technique a wonderful surprise awaits you. The strength created through many of the standing-leg routines will bring with it renewed balance and poise. Additionally, as your balance improves so will your quality of exercise, as you focus more on technique.

STRENGTH TRAINING

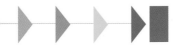

When it comes to strength training a comment I hear more than any other is 'I don't want to get big muscles'. Why is it that women resist weights? Perhaps we have conjured up an image of burly over-pumped men groaning their way through a gruelling weights session in a steamy, sweaty gym. Or maybe you plucked up the courage in the past to join a gym but were ill-advised on the use of the equipment and as a result have built up muscle in the wrong places.

Whatever your anxieties surrounding strength training, I aim to dispel them. It is very difficult to build big muscles. You would have to train like a body builder, almost every day and with very heavy weights. With a pair of light to medium hand-held weights and a clear understanding of technique, you can totally transform your body. I have, and so have many of my clients. If you are not familiar with working out with weights, welcome to a workout that is going to stop your muscles from sagging and being untoned to being taut and toned. If you have used weights in the past with little success, your technique was probably not up to scratch. By learning the correct principles for strength training you will understand exactly where you have gone wrong in the past.

Long-term weight loss

The key to permanent weight loss is to increase muscle mass so that you burn extra calories all day long.

We've stepped, salsa'd and done high impact. We've got the cowboy boots out for line dancing. We've done kick boxing, tae bo, and now it's yoga and pilates. Whilst each of these methods of getting fit have something valuable to offer, researchers have concluded that the key to long-term weight loss is to engage in strength-training exercises. Daniel Gastelu, a pioneer in performance nutrition, backs this up with conviction. 'Weight training stands out as the single best method for ensuring that weight loss comes from fat stores and not from hard-won muscle tissue. Why? Because aerobic training simply does not build muscle to the extent that weight training does. In fact, aerobic training alone tends to reduce lean-body mass and cause a drop in resting metabolic rate.'

REAL WOMEN
and the Jenergy Way

'I was a complete fitness nut when I first met Jenni, a keen runner as well as attending aerobic classes every week. I decided to go and try one of her classes. The neat, toned bodies ranging from early thirties to early sixties were profoundly noticeable in her class. The second thing that struck me was whilst I had hardly broken a bead of sweat, the rest of the class, including Jenni, were drenched in perspiration. "Perhaps I am just too fit," I thought. A year later I have a very different perspective on those first thoughts. Jenni took me aside one day and questioned me about my training. I told her I ran and did lots of high impact classes. "What about strength training?" she asked. My admission of being able to do 20 push-ups and any amount of sit-ups failed to impress her.

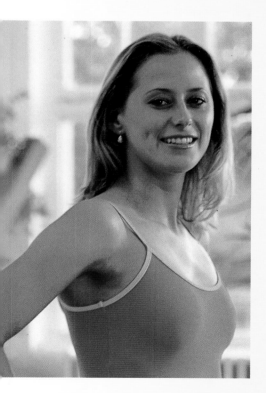

She explained the importance of adding strength training to my programme but, more importantly, she stressed that my quality of movement was poor and that was the reason I was finding the classes so simple. From that day onwards I attended two classes a week and stood right in the front so that I could start to understand her technique. I decreased my running and stopped aerobic classes altogether. In addition to going down one dress size, my body fat has gone from 27–21% in a year. Interestingly, my weight has remained the same. I feel sexier and healthier being toned, whereas before I was fit, but untoned.'

SARKA KARTAKOVA

Attending aerobic classes or jogging will certainly get your cardiovascular system fit. Unfortunately it will do little to increase your strength. Once you add resistance training to your programme there will be a noted change in your body composition and posture. The reason for this is that muscles require extra calories to service and maintain them. Our resting metabolic rate (RMR) is defined as the pace at which calories are burned at rest. This is closely linked to the amount of muscle in your body. The loss of muscle slows down your RMR, thus fewer calories are burned. The key to successful long-term weight loss is to understand the importance of increasing the amount of muscle in your body.

Every pound of muscle added to the body burns about 35 extra calories per day, or about 3–4 pounds of fat every year.

As your RMR goes up, more calories will be burned during all activities, including sitting, lying down and sleeping. The less muscle you have, the lower your metabolism and the easier it is to gain weight. For this reason, it is important to set long-term goals for yourself.

Benefits of having a firm, toned body

Besides looking great, feeling younger and sexier and being able to wear great clothes, you will also benefit from decreased fat, increased bone density, improved functional strength, posture and muscle balance. Many researchers believe that strength training can help prevent and even reverse some of the physical effects of ageing.

'Burn more calories, even when you're not exercising.'

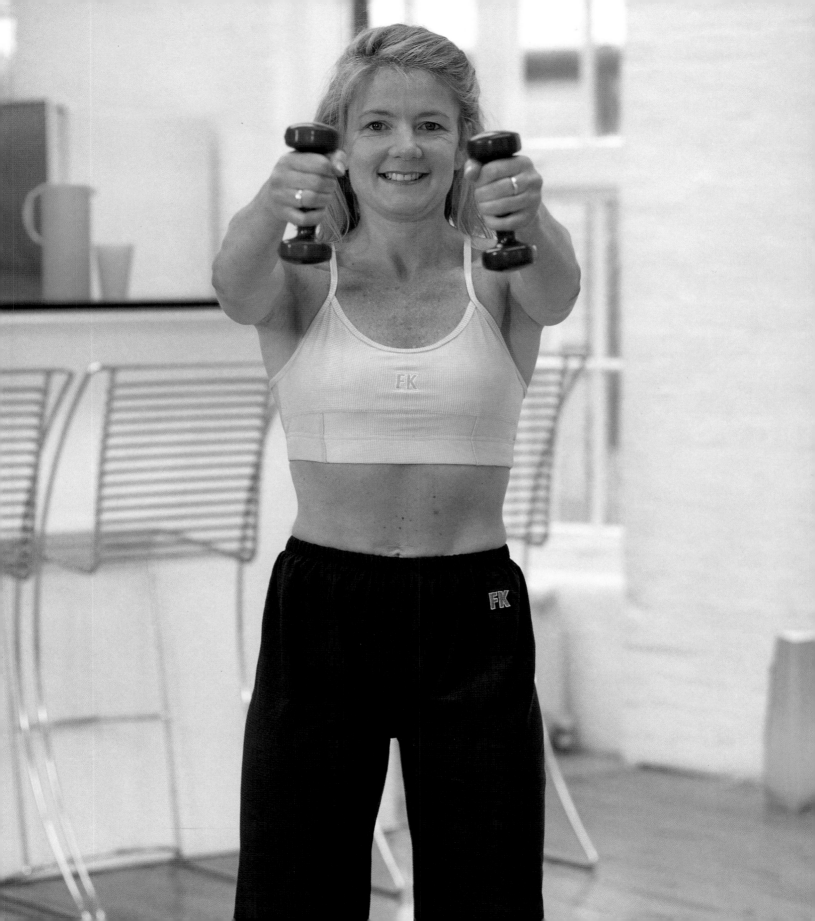

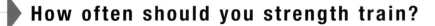

How often should you strength train?

How soon do you want to see results? Douglas Brooks says significant gains in strength and muscular endurance can be achieved with just two exercise sessions per week. This means at least 10 exercises that target all of the major muscle groups. At least one set of 8–12 repetitions, completed to fatigue, should be performed to gain health benefits. This is not daunting. With proper planning you could design a strength-training routine, which could be completed in 15 minutes. To make it even more time efficient, you could switch regularly from the upper to the lower body keeping the intensity up, and thereby stimulating further fat release. You could even work the upper and lower body simultaneously, as some of my exercises in this book will demonstrate. My personal advice, in conjunction with the exercises, would be to strength train two to four times a week. Here are some guidelines.

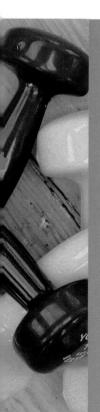

Strength training guidelines

- When working out with light weights for general toning, strength train up to four times a week. Do 12–16 reps, 2–3 sets.

- When working out with heavier weights, strength train twice a week. Do 2–3 sets.

- Choose one or two exercises for each muscle group and do them at each session.

- Work all the abdominal muscles three to four times a week.

- Choose four or five lower-body exercises and do them four to six times a week. Stretch afterwards.

- If your technique is poor – results will be poor.

REAL WOMEN
and the Jenergy Way

'I am a business woman with a hectic schedule. I deal with the public on a regular basis which means that looking smart and feeling fit are paramount to me being able to cope with the welter of diverse situations my job brings with it. Having joined gym after gym I have found it almost impossible to meet the high standards I have encountered whilst on business trips to the US and it has frustrated me immensely as time is my most valuable asset.

Then a chance meeting through a mutual friend brought Jenni into my life. Jenni helped me stock up my home gym with equipment that I can use when training on my own, such as a treadmill and free weights. I found Jenni's knowledge beyond reproach and decided that I wanted her to oversee my

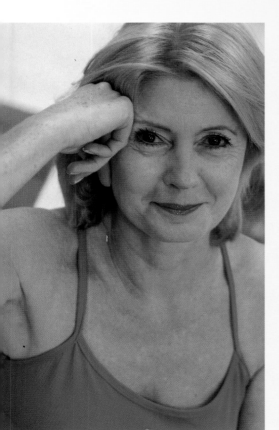

training once a week. My programme was totally revamped based on my goals, what I wanted to achieve and my problem areas. Over time I have begun to understand how important it is to have a planned and focused workout. Added to this, I have mastered the correct technique for working each and every muscle correctly, making it easy to maintain my fit and toned body. More importantly, having the knowledge to train correctly has meant that I only need to work out twice a week.'

MARGARET LEVIN

A WOMAN-ONLY APPROACH

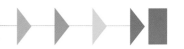

Train with the Jenergy 'woman-only-approach' and achieve a beautifully sculpted body. We are women and we want to look like women, and yet men devise many of our exercise programmes. Men have different goals to women. The question 'does my bum look big in this?' is one surely to have passed many women's lips at some stage. Basically, men and women have entirely different goals when it comes to the shape of their bodies. Most men want big arms and chest, whilst women would rather have smaller, toned arms with firm breasts that don't sag. Men want a six-pack stomach whilst most women want to be able to zip up their jeans with ease. Men want to look more masculine and women want to enhance their feminine curves.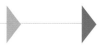

Women have a genetic predisposition for storing fat on the hips, thighs and buttocks, and their bodies are designed to store fat far more efficiently than a man's. This is very obviously to prepare a woman's body for a nine-month supply of fat to protect an unborn child. In simple terms, a woman's body will accumulate enough fat so that there's always a 'reserve tank' of fuel in case of a famine. The principles outlined here place focus on the lower body, regarded as a woman's major problem area, and the exercises are specifically designed to be performed frequently using little or no weight. This consistent over training (from four to six times per week) gives the lower body no option but to slim down and tone up.

These physical differences alone should make it clear that men and women should train differently. A number of women clients who had previously worked with die-hard men trainers were sceptical about changing onto my programme. They had come to see me because they felt they were bulking up in the wrong places. However, having spent hours in a gym, working out with heavy weights and leg machines and then being told they could achieve a great shape with just their own body weight and a few dumbbells was difficult for them to comprehend. After spending a few months on the new routine they all slimmed down and felt more feminine about their shape. Following a planned, focused routine to suit the unique needs of a woman's body was all they needed to do. These are the changes they made:

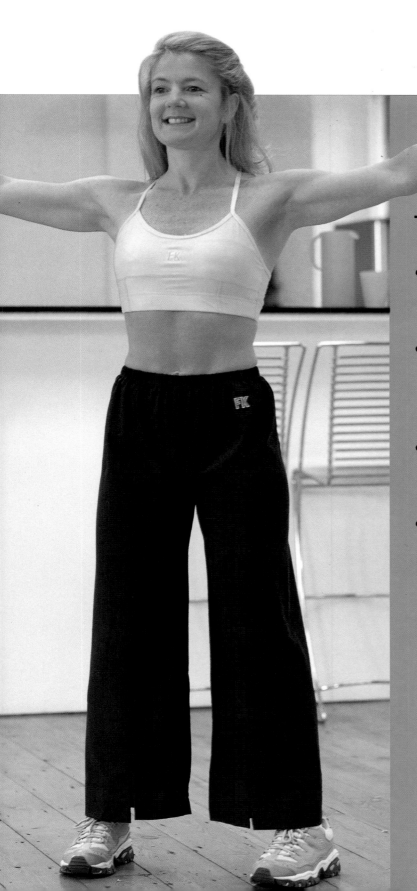

The changes they made

- To encourage fat burning they walked/ jogged for 30–40 minutes, three to four times a week at the right intensity.

- More emphasis was placed on working the triceps, backs of the shoulders and back muscles with light to medium weights, and high repetitions.

- The lower body was trained with more frequency – up to six times a week, to start off with.

- The abdominals were worked at every session.

The ultimate success of their changes came as a result of implementing the Jenergy strength-training techniques into each and every exercise.

My approach

Although I have a great success rate with both men and women when it comes to achieving their fitness goals, my real talent lies with helping women achieve their personal best. Spending years as a gymnast helped me form the basis of my woman-only approach. Much of the training done by gymnasts is based on working with their own body weight. The strength, balance, and coordination skills required by gymnasts do not come from working on gym machines. Their upper-body strength comes from working on the parallel bars and the rings using their own body strength. Their lower-body strength and balance comes from hours of standing-leg routines which recruit more than one muscle group at a time, creating lean, toned and lengthened muscles through the lower body.

In addition to being a gymnast, I also had the wonderful experience of teaching aqua aerobics in Perth, Australia. As this was a relatively new concept I set about creating a class of my own. Very soon I was teaching all the leg routines on the side of the pool, enabling the ladies to follow me. Before long, the firmest, leanest legs and buttocks I have ever had, started to emerge. This experience and my time as a gymnast were enough ammunition for me to start developing and teaching my principles all over the world. With years of hands-on experience working with women, I have designed the perfect concept along with a dictionary of exercises aimed to completely re-shape those stubborn areas most women encounter.

My technique aims to create strength, balance and beautifully streamlined legs and buttocks with a fit, firm and feminine-looking upper body.

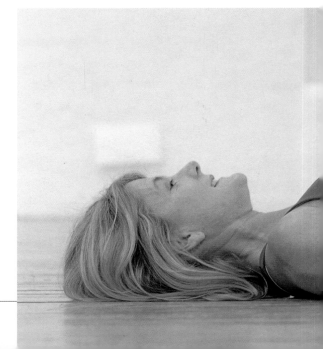

Lower-body principles

We are all familiar with traditional floor work exercises for the lower body. Let's see how this floor work compares to a more dynamic method of training. Take the side-lying leg lifts. Although you are certainly isolating the outer thigh muscles, the floor is supporting the rest of the body. Now take the same exercise and perform it in a standing position. Not only are you recruiting many more muscles through the lower body, but you are also having to use the abdominals as a constant source of support. This functional exercise, as it is commonly known, simply gets the task done in half the time. In the same way, by sitting on a leg-extension machine, the entire body is being supported and only the front thigh muscle is being worked. When time is an all-important factor we want to make our workouts as efficient as possible, which is exactly what the Jenergy lower-body principles do.

Many of the standing-leg routines challenge the muscles to really work hard against gravity. By placing resistance on the upward part of most leg routines you will be achieving this.

We are women, we want to look like women.

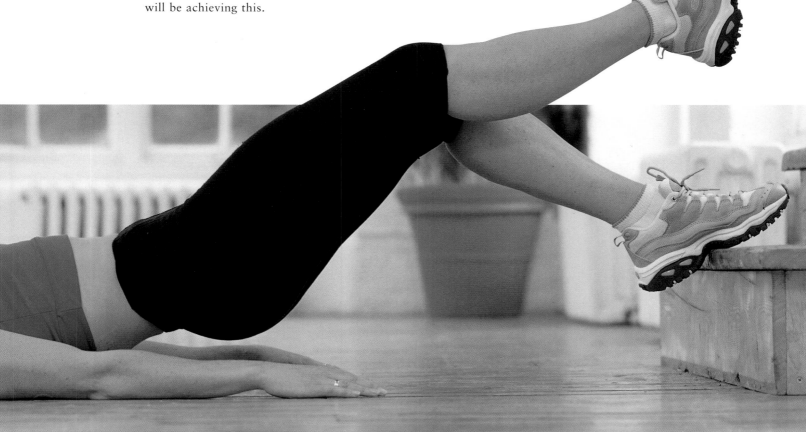

MAXIMISE YOUR FAT BLAST

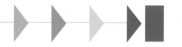

We are now fully aware of the importance of strength training for long-term weight loss by increasing muscle mass and boosting metabolism. Let us not confuse this with fat-burning exercise. If your goal is to burn calories, stick to cardiovascular training. Per hour, you're going to use up at least twice as many calories doing something cardio as you would strength training. Which should you do to lose weight? Both – at least two to three times a week.

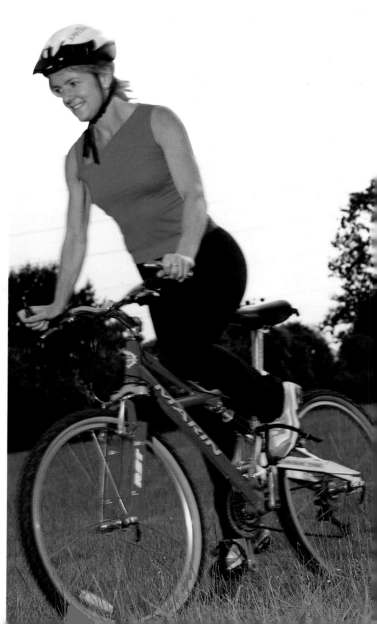

Benefits

- Decreases body fat stores.

- Decreases total cholesterol.

- Decreases symptoms of depression, anxiety and tension.

- Decreases resting heart rate.

- Reduces blood pressure.

- Increases heart function.

- Increases blood flow to active muscles.

- Increases lung capacity.

- Increases mobilisation and utilisation of fat.

REAL WOMEN
and the Jenergy Way

'One of the best pieces of advice Jenni gave me was how easy it is to fit exercise into your life if it is planned and focused. My life is hectic to say the least, having to get up most mornings at 4am and then appear fresh and happy on morning TV. I used to come home in the afternoon, exhausted, and, before I met Jenni, the thought of exercise was the last thing on my mind.

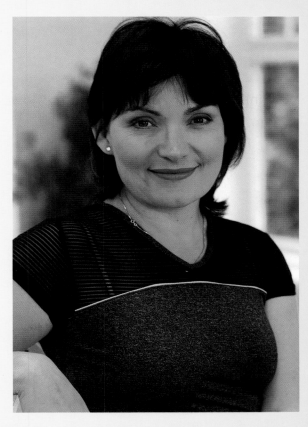

When Jenni explained that just three, 30-minute power walks up and down the hills near my home would be enough to keep my weight down and increase my energy levels, I was surprised. The walks became part of my weekly routine. My energy levels drastically improved and it was great to have that energy for my family at the end of the day. However, my weight did not seem to change drastically. Then one day Jenni came out with me and explained that I was not walking at the right intensity. She taught me to work with a heart rate monitor, keeping the intensity within a certain range. Well, what a difference. The weight started to fall off after that. It's a great form of exercise for me as I can do it anywhere provided I can make the commitment to do it three times a week. I now feel sure my weight will never go up again, and more importantly, I now know how simple it all is once you are told the guidelines.'

LORRAINE KELLY

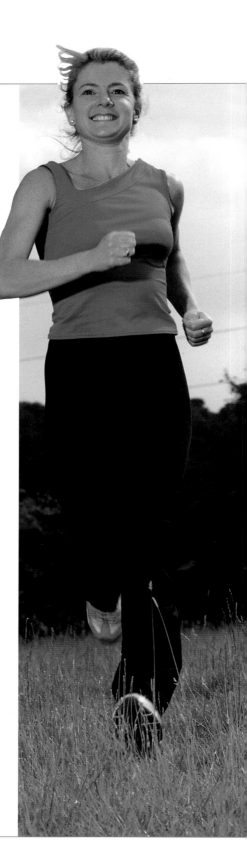

Aerobic exercise

When we hear the word aerobic, we tend to think of a room full of slinkily clad bodies all moving in time to an upbeat song. This is because aerobics has become such a widely used word and we inevitably think of it in that context. But, what can aerobic exercise do for you? If you are one of those people who has decided to try and improve your quality of life, aerobic exercises are an excellent starting point.

Cardio-respiratory fitness refers to the health and function of the heart, lungs and circulatory system, which is brought about by aerobic activity. When working out aerobically you require more than the normal consumption of oxygen. Aerobic simply means working with oxygen. There are a number of activities that are aerobic. These include walking, jogging, running, step and aerobic classes, swimming, cycling, rowing, hiking and racket sports. When you work out aerobically the main fuel comes from fat, along with carbohydrates, so aerobic exercise forces the fat cells to release fat. By doing this on a regular basis your fat-releasing enzyme is forced to release fat and in turn your fat cells are going to decrease.

By taking the following four factors into consideration you can work out your aerobic programme:

Your aerobic programme
- Determine which exercise is best for you.
- Decide the length of each session.
- Decide how often you can do it.
- Exercise at the right intensity.

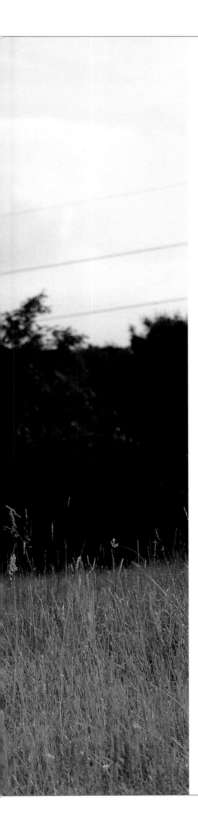

Exercise selection

You are now ready to decide what is best for you. Obviously, you have to be capable of taking on the activity of your choice. It is no use deciding that you will go cycling 10 miles every other day if you have dodgy knees. Likewise, you would not choose swimming if you still use arm bands. Be realistic about what you are capable of. Next, you need to look at your available time. If you work in the city, then there is no point joining the local gym where you live, because chances are you will never get there. It is important, in the long term, that you select an aerobic activity that you will enjoy. There is no point in doing something that holds little interest for you.

Finally, you will need to decide whether your chosen activity requires equipment and facilities. Most fitness clubs will have all the aerobic facilities available and some even have swimming pools and racket courts. Many activities require little or no equipment at all, and often it is better to start out this way and then invest time and money when you are convinced that you want to continue.

Cross-country skiing and squash are rated as the top calorie burners. As cross-country skiing is not readily available to everyone, a cross-country ski trainer which simulates the same motions is the next best thing. Hill climbing is another huge energy user – an eight-hour day with brief rests will burn an average of 4,000 calories. Swimming is also a fantastic calorie-burning exercise, although it doesn't burn off as much fat as weight-bearing exercises. Fitness researcher Wayne Westcott says studies have shown that people who swim aren't as lean as those who do activities like running or cycling. However, it is still a great way to use your whole body and especially beneficial if used in a cross-training routine.

My personal recommendation for an aerobic activity would be one in which exercise intensity is easily sustained with little variability in the heart rate: walking, jogging, running, swimming, aerobic classes and cross-country skiing, and the various aerobic machines on offer in the fitness clubs. Some of these activities are achievable without the use of equipment and/or facilities, and you can complete them within 45 minutes.

Exercise duration

Over the past decade the duration of aerobic activity has been much the subject of debate and we have seen quite a number of changes being made in this area. Initially, the guidelines were to do 20 minutes of aerobic exercise, three times per week for the most effective way to burn fat or increase your lean-body tissue. Then more research came out to suggest that we needed to increase the duration of the aerobic activity to 30–45 minutes, three times per week. This was overwhelming or simply too much for many people who, as a result, gave up or did not even start. Now we have been advised to accumulate 30 minutes of any exercise that is aerobic throughout the day, such as a 5-minute walk to the bus stop, with a 10-minute lunchtime swim, and walking up and down two flights of stairs in a day. The experts are even suggesting that doing 10 minutes of exercise per day can be of great benefit. This is good news for us because it is encouraging to know that every little bit helps. If you find that occasionally there are days when you simply cannot fit 30–45 minutes in, all in one go, then breaking the aerobic section up into two sessions is just as beneficial. In this situation, you could do 15 minutes on the stair master first thing in the morning, and maybe fit a power walk in at lunchtime. The choice is yours.

However, for best results I would strongly recommend you aim to complete your 30–45 minutes in one session. Once it is done there is no need for excuses as to why you haven't been able to do it. This 30–45 minutes excludes the warm up and cool down sessions. Be sure to leave time for these.

The key to fat and calorie burning is understanding the link between intensity and weight loss.

After just 20 minutes of aerobic exercise your fat-releasing enzymes have kicked in and are releasing fat, which is being burnt up for energy. In addition the body continues to burn fat at a higher level for up to 36 hours after aerobic exercise. If you have chosen to walk or run, getting yourself out of the front door is probably the hardest part of the decision. However, once a regular routine has been established it becomes easier. Spending 45 minutes on one piece of cardiovascular equipment in the gym can become quite mundane. My suggestion is to move around the different machines on offer. For example, spend 10 minutes on the treadmill, then 5 minutes on the rowing machine, then another 10 minutes on the stair master, and finish up with 10 minutes on the bike. Each time mix it around by spending more time on some machines than others and by changing the order. Walk in with a focus and avoid getting caught up in a conversation which will distract you.

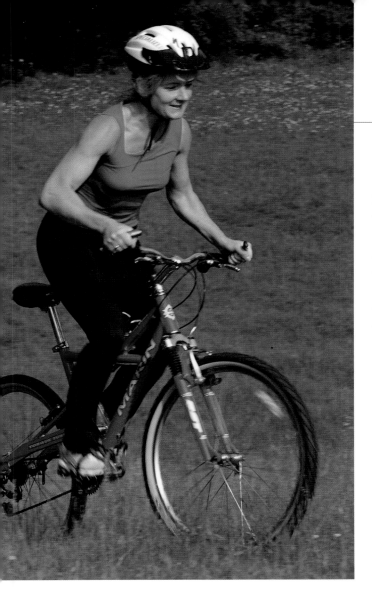

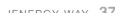

Exercise frequency

How quickly you want to see changes in your body shape should answer the question of how often to exercise. I have had a great success rate with a frequency of three to five times per week. Research shows that the difference between exercising aerobically twice a week and exercising three times a week is quite significant. If someone is only able to see me once or twice a week, I am quite strict about ensuring they try to get at least one more aerobic session in. This may sound a lot to you at first, but if you think about it realistically it is only one and a half hours per week, broken up into three half-hour sessions. There really is no reason to exercise aerobically more than five times per week. When you start training at this sort of level, you really are expending a great amount of energy, and if you are not replacing the energy with a huge amount of calories, we begin to see problems with the metabolic rate. However, for those of you just beginning an exercise programme or trying to lose weight, I suggest you do at least four to five aerobic sessions per week for the best results, and this will also encourage you to continue, especially when you notice how quickly the weight is dropping off.

I strongly recommend that you don't put your aerobic exercise off to the last minute, which is why it is not a bad idea to try and fit it in first thing in the morning – that way you've done it and there are no excuses that have to be made later on. Understandably, many of us are not morning people and there is no evidence to suggest that exercising in the morning is more beneficial than at any other time of the day. Exercising first thing in the morning has the positive advantage of making you feel energised for the whole day, and therefore positive about all your other goals or achievements for the day. Somehow, sitting down for breakfast, after you have been out exercising for an hour, seems so well earned.

Exercise intensity

Have you ever been in an aerobics class and half way through the instructor has stopped the class and asked everyone to take their pulse rate? This was to try and gauge exercise intensity. My experience is that most people don't have any idea how, why or what they are trying to achieve when taking their pulse rate.

Intensity of aerobic exercise has been much the topic of debate in the past few years and we are now seeing a shift in focus on intensity of exercise, from the traditional Target Heart Rate Chart, which used to prescribe aerobic exercise within a target zone of 60–90% of age-predicted maximal heart rate (Age–PMHR), to a newly developed Heart Rate Guide showing that even small increases above Resting Heart Rate may be beneficial to health, while greater increases can provide both health and fitness benefits. Basically, there is still a high percentage of inactive people out there, many of whom believe that unless exercise is very strenuous and intense it is not worth doing. Exercise does not have to be vigorous to be beneficial, and even modest amounts of physical activity, such as walking and gardening, can improve overall health and increase weight loss. However, intensity of exercise is an all-important factor to consider if weight loss or increased fitness is your goal. This has been a key factor in helping many of my clients lose those last ten pounds. Very often I see the same faces with the same bodies in the gym month after month. That's because they are putting no effort into the intensity of their exercise. They're either worried about ruining their hair with perspiration, or they are chatting. Perhaps they simply do not understand the important link between intensity and weight loss.

Aerobic exercise should be done at the right intensity for maximum fat burning.

One of the best ways to monitor exercise intensity is with a heart rate monitor. This is basically a device which provides you with immediate feedback on the level of intensity of whichever exercise you are involved in. A transmitter belt worn around the chest transfers the heartbeat signal to a receiver, which is in the form of a wristwatch. Once my clients have reached a certain level of fitness, I encourage them to increase the intensity, as this overall increase will have the double benefit of increasing their fitness level, as well as burning more calories and therefore more fat.

For those of you who don't have a heart rate monitor, you can learn to take your own pulse rate by placing two fingers gently over the carotid artery located on either side of your neck. Once you feel your pulse, begin counting for six seconds. Simply multiply that figure by 10 or add a zero on the end to determine your heart rate. For example, if you counted 12 beats during a six-second count starting from 0, then your pulse rate is 120. After practising a few times it becomes easier. To work out what the best intensity for weight loss or increased fitness levels is, use the following formula:

First determine your own maximum heart rate. Maximum heart rate means the number of beats per minute in a situation where even if intensity was increased, the rate would not increase any further. You can estimate maximum heart rate from the following formula:

220 – age (in years) = maximum heart rate

For example, the maximum heart rate for a 30-year old woman will be: 220 – 30 = 190 beats per minute. The rate that uses the greatest expenditure of energy consumption from fat metabolism is 60–70% of the maximum heart rate. Exercise performed at this intensity forces the muscle cells to derive most of their energy from fat reserves. As you get fitter, start working closer to the higher end of the weight-loss range, and for longer.

Knowing how to take your pulse rate to gauge exercise intensity is crucial to weight loss and increased fitness.

Age	Maximum heart rate (beats/min)	Range for weight loss (beats/min)	Aerobic training zone (beats/min)
20	200	120–140	140–160
30	190	114–133	133–152
40	180	108–126	126–144
50	170	102–119	119–136
60	160	96–112	112–128

Now let me undo a little myth that seemed to have been blown out of all proportion in the early 1990s. Everyone seemed to be doing this funny hip wiggle walk and apparently they were burning major fat. I even remember getting hooked on this whole debate of fat burning myself. Exercisers were being told to slow down and work at a lower intensity to burn more fat. And slowing down they were!

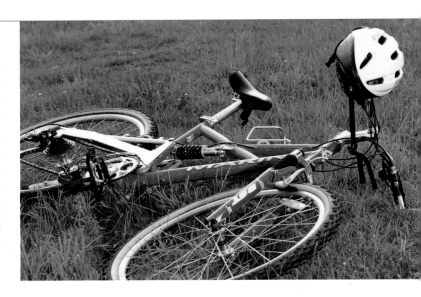

Fat burning

Let's clarify this whole 'fat burning' issue. If you are starting out on an exercise programme and you are relatively unfit, it is advisable to start out at a lower intensity and the primary source of energy will come from fat. Pushing the intensity up too quickly on an untrained body will push it into a semi-state of emergency, which will cause the primary fuel to come from carbohydrates. However, as your fitness level improves, it is extremely important to work well within your fat-burning range. This way you will be utilising a greater percentage of total calories and therefore a greater percentage of fat. As you get fitter move up to a higher level of intensity to maximise your fat burning and, provided the systems have modified and adapted, you will continue to burn a greater percentage of fat.

As your fitness level improves, work at the top end of your fat-burning range and higher.

When researchers compared high-intensity exercise with endurance training, they found the more vigorous workout produced greater fat loss. They concluded that vigorous exercise (about 70% of maximal heart rate) for 45–60 minutes caused an increase in fat-burning enzymes, a greater rise in resting metabolic rate and therefore greater weight loss, in the long run. To maximise fat burning, the key is to work as long as possible at as high an intensity as possible in order to maximise calorie burning. This can be implemented as you get fitter.

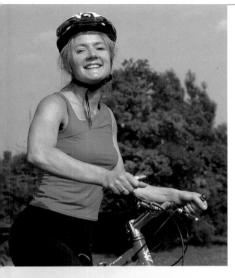

Aerobic guidelines

- Select one or more aerobic activities of your choice.

- Exercise aerobically three to five times per week.

- Aim to do a minimum of 30–45 minutes in each session.

- If you cannot fit 30–45 minutes into each session, then split it up.

- Work out at the right intensity during each session.

- Vary your workouts often and cross train.

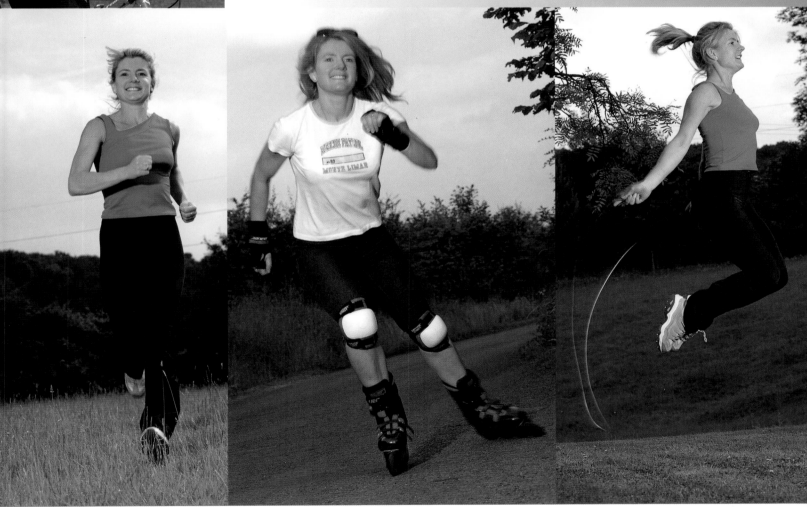

The EXERCISES

- *Muscle groups and Equipment*

- *Warming up*

- *Super-toned arms*

- *Beautiful back and posture*

- *Look behind*

- *Fab abs forever*

- *Stretching*

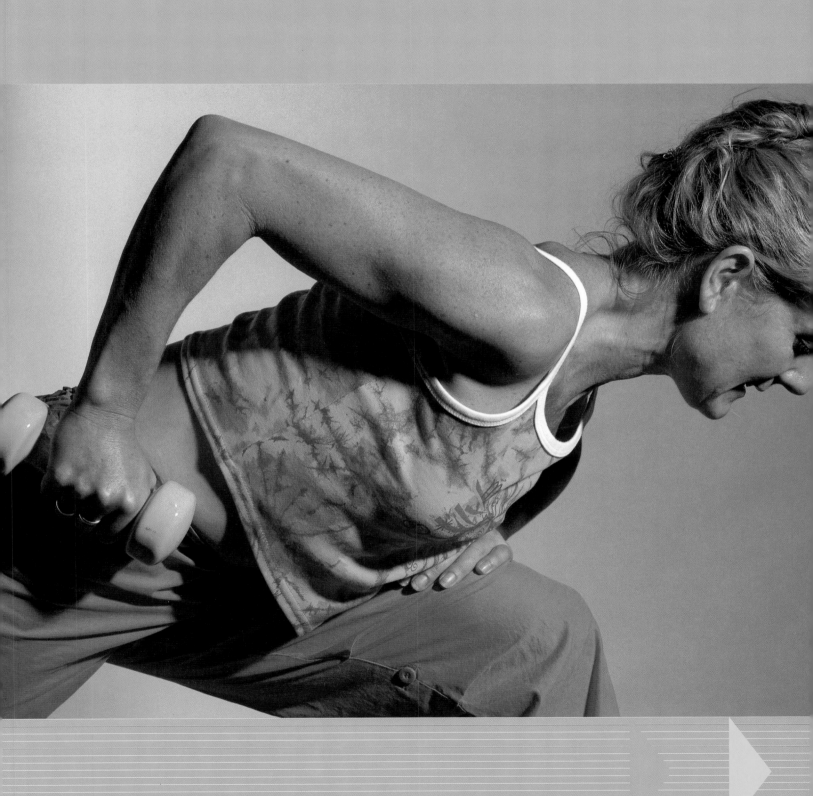

MUSCLES

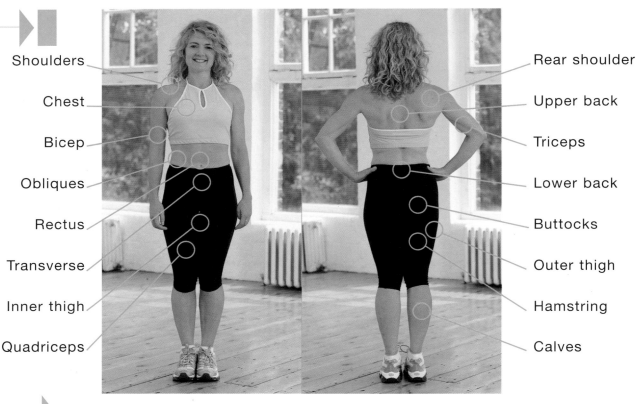

Shoulders
Chest
Bicep
Obliques
Rectus
Transverse
Inner thigh
Quadriceps

Rear shoulder
Upper back
Triceps
Lower back
Buttocks
Outer thigh
Hamstring
Calves

Muscles in balance

Our bodies naturally produce some muscles stronger than others. For example, the front thigh muscles tend to be 33% stronger than the opposing back thigh muscles. Many women tend to only work their abdominals and buttocks, in the same way men will over train their chests and not their legs. By over training certain muscles at the expense of others, we can disturb the natural balance between the strength and flexibility of those muscles and muscle imbalances..

Although the majority of these exercises have been designed especially for the unique needs of a woman's body, it is important that you work through all the exercises to ensure that no muscle is neglected, thereby avoiding any joint-related problems.

Breathing

Breathing correctly will execute more power through each move. Holding your breath or not concentrating on breathing will tense the muscles. Technique declines when working with tense muscles – they will contract far better from a relaxed state produced by proper breathing. When exercising aim to exhale on the effort, which is the more difficult part of the move. Inhale on the return part of the exercise.

EQUIPMENT

Skipping rope

Add variety to your workouts by skipping. One of the best all round exercises and you can take the rope anywhere. Invest in a speed rope.

Tubing and bands

These add fantastic resistance to leg routines and both are great for working the upper body – a bonus if you are travelling as you can get a full body workout. I wouldn't leave home without mine!

The step

A useful piece of equipment but not absolutely necessary. If you do not have a step then use your staircase. The step acts as a useful prop with many of the lying down workouts.

Exercise ball

This is one of the most versatile pieces of equipment to have. By constantly having to keep the ball stable, the central girdle is contracted throughout most exercises building great strength and balance through this section of the body. It is advisable to be careful with some of the exercises and to perfect them off the ball first. If you are of average height then get a 63cm ball. If you are much taller then go for the 75cm ball.

Dumbbells

They've been around forever and still hold a prime spot in the world of fitness equipment. Invest in a pair of 1kg, 2kg and 3kg weights. My favourite choice would be the vinyl dipped dumbbells.

WARMING UP

Benefits of a proper warm up

- Increased heart rate.

- Increased blood pressure.

- Increased oxygen consumption.

- Dilation of the blood vessels.

- Prevents injury.

Many of us are aware of the importance of warming up before exercising but often tend to ignore this component by rushing straight into our routine. This is not advisable – besides the immense benefits of warming up, injury could result.

To warm up correctly, prepare the body for the exercise to follow by utilising the same muscle groups, followed by a few stretching moves. Rushing a warm up causes lactic acid to build up, leading to fatigue early in your workout. Since we are not aiming to increase our flexibility at this stage, the stretches should remain fluid-like and not be held for too long. Experts agree it is best to stretch after you exercise because the muscles are warm and pliable.

If you are planning on doing a power walk followed by some strength-training exercises, a safe warm up would be about 7–10 minutes. These would be followed by some of the warm-up stretches shown.

Walking

Start off with movements such as marching on the spot or walking slowly.

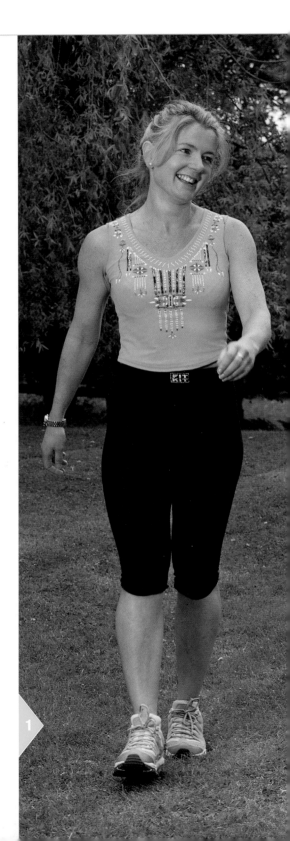

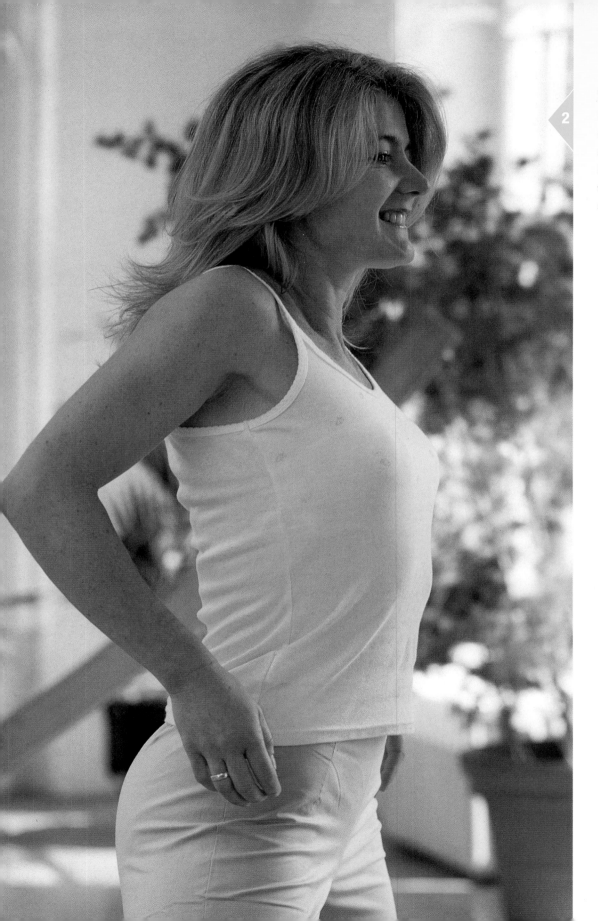

Shoulder Rolls

Relax your arms and bring your shoulders up towards your ears and then roll them back by bringing your shoulder blades together. Continue circling your shoulders about 8 times.

The Spine

This is a good preparatory move for any exercise or sport because it stretches and mobilises the back. Stand with your feet a little further than shoulder-distance apart, knees bent. Keeping your lower body stationary, round your spine out without letting your torso drop forwards. Release and repeat 8 times.

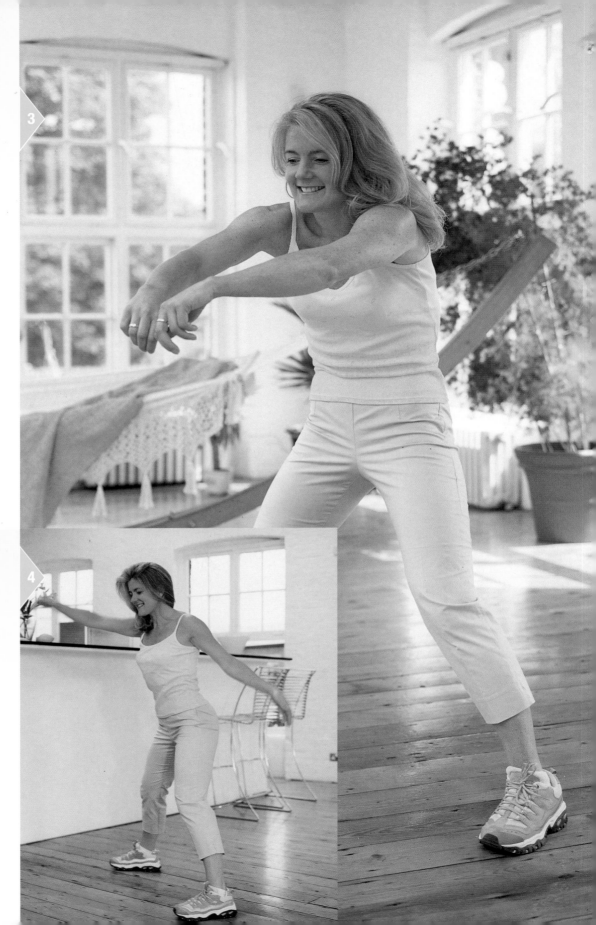

Front Crawl

This move recruits more muscle groups through the back and arms. Stand with your feet a little further than shoulder-distance apart, knees bent. Keeping your lower body stationary, bring your right arm behind, over and in front of you. Repeat on your left side (as in the front crawl stroke). Repeat 4 times on each side, alternating.

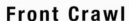

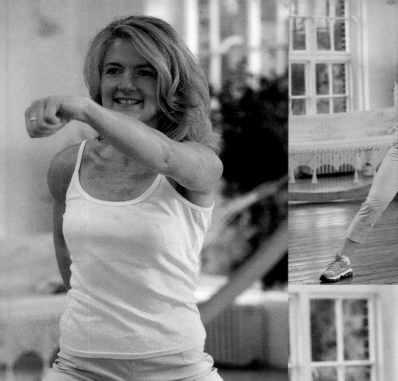

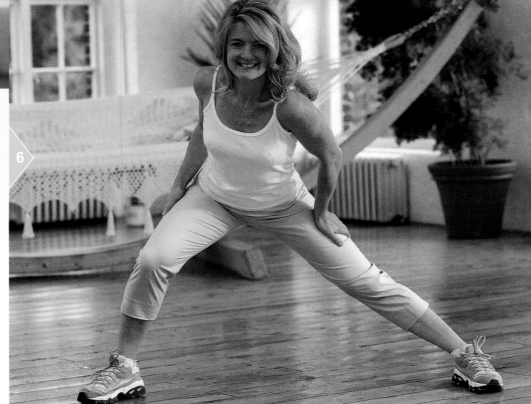

Side Stretch

Stand with your feet shoulder-distance apart, knees slightly bent. Reaching your right arm diagonally up and across your body, try to keep your hips stationary and pull out of the lats. Reach alternate arms across in a continuous routine. Repeat 8 times on each side.

Side to Side Lunges

Stand with your feet a little further than shoulder-distance apart, feet turned out slightly. Shift your body weight gently from right to left, making sure the knee does not extend over the ankle.

Warm-up sequence

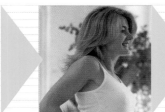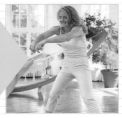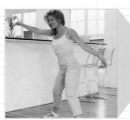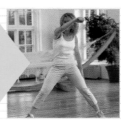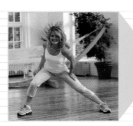

SUPER-TONED ARMS

As women we tend to be more obsessed with the state of our lower body and stomach muscles. However, there is nothing more depressing than having to cover your arms with a cardigan on a warm day because they are unsightly. Many women avoid training their upper body because they are afraid of building up too much muscle. As I have already mentioned, it would take seriously heavy weights and hours of training to get big, bulky muscles.

This programme has been specifically designed to help you attain lean, toned arms without any bulk. Working with light to medium weights, high reps and perfect technique your arms will soon take on a look that will make you proud to go sleeveless even on the chilliest of days.

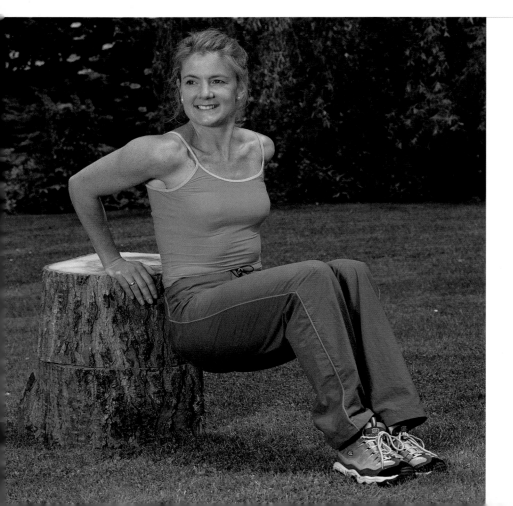

Triceps

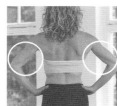

These muscles tend to be relatively weak in most women and are one of the first muscles on a woman's body to sag. Because they are not used enough in everyday activities, it is important that you get to grips with them and work them regularly.

Choose two of the following exercises at every session and work your triceps 2–3 times a week.

Dips

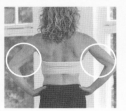

Equipment: ball/bench
15 reps, 2 sets

This is one of the most effective ways of doing a triceps dip. The legs and abdominals are used as a constant source of stabilisation making it an advanced exercise that can also be done on the end of a chair, a bath or with the use of the ball.

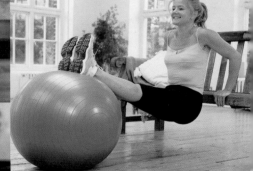

Watch Out!

● Keep your elbows close to the centre of your body.
● Do not lock your elbows on the lift.
● Do not let your shoulders shrug up.

Squeeze your shoulder blades together and slowly drop your buttocks towards the floor until your upper arms are almost parallel to the ceiling. Straighten your arms and repeat.

1

Sitting on the end of a chair with your hands facing forwards, rest your feet on the floor. Lift your buttocks off the chair, keeping your abs contracted and your back straight.

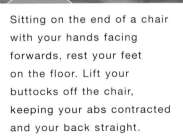

2

Triceps Extension on a Ball

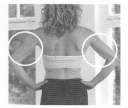

Equipment: 1–2kg weight
12–15 reps, 2–3 sets

In addition to working the triceps, you are using the hamstring and abdominals to keep the rest of the body supported. This can be done lying on the floor.

Watch Out!

- Keep your upper arms stationary. They are not invited to the party!
- Keep your elbows close to your head.
- Squeeze for a split second at the top of the move.

Keeping your upper arms stationary, bend your elbows and slowly lower your hands to either side of your head. Lift the weights up again, without locking your elbows. Hold for a split second and lower again.

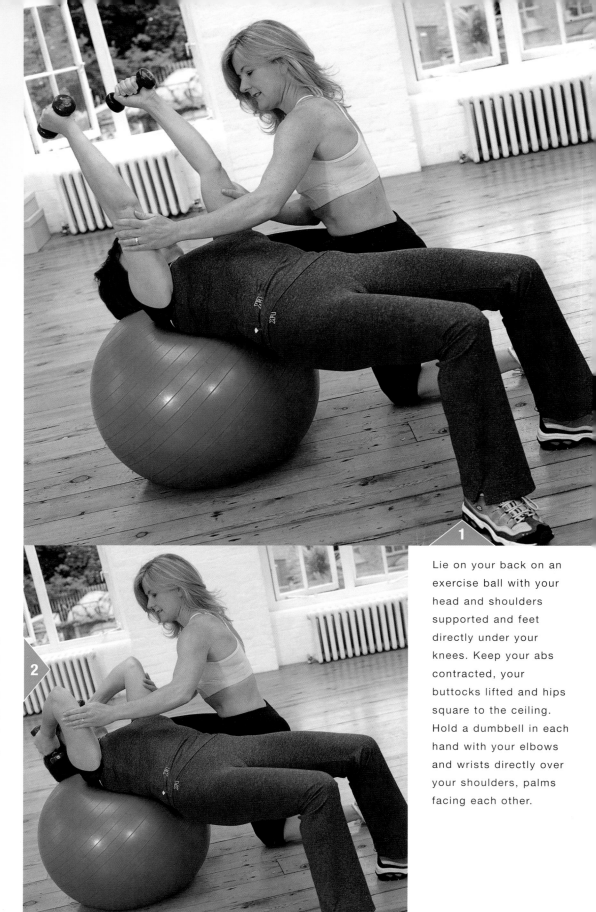

Lie on your back on an exercise ball with your head and shoulders supported and feet directly under your knees. Keep your abs contracted, your buttocks lifted and hips square to the ceiling. Hold a dumbbell in each hand with your elbows and wrists directly over your shoulders, palms facing each other.

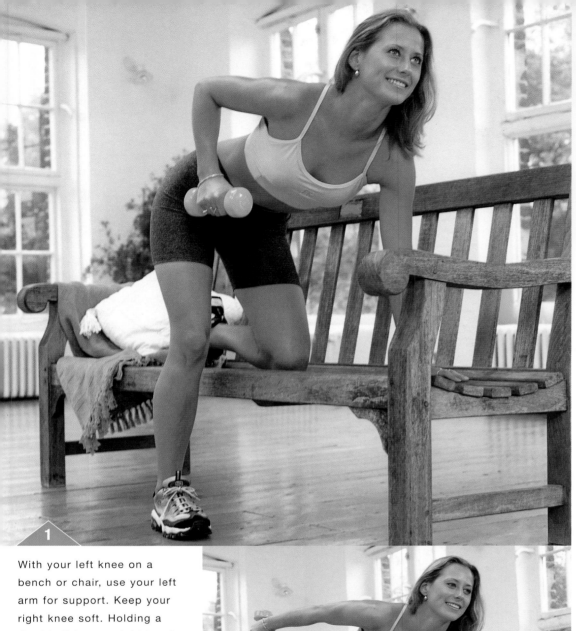

Single Arm Triceps Extension

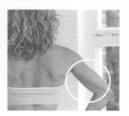

**Equipment: 2–3kg weight
15 reps, 2 sets**

This exercise can be done with a slightly heavier weight – and slower, since only one arm is being worked at a time. Sort out those flabby underarm bits!

Watch Out!
- Use control and not momentum.
- Keep your wrist straight.
- Keep your upper arm stationary.

1 With your left knee on a bench or chair, use your left arm for support. Keep your right knee soft. Holding a dumbbell in your right hand, lift the upper arm up until it is parallel to the floor.

2 Keeping your abs contracted and your back straight, extend the weight out until the whole arm is almost parallel to the floor, without locking your elbow. Hold for a split second and release slowly. Repeat on the other side.

Double Arm Triceps Extension

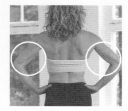

Equipment: 1–2kg weight
15–20 reps, 2 sets

Executed with perfect technique, this high frequency, light-weighted exercise will quickly tone up the backs of your arms.

Watch Out!

- Keep your back straight.
- Keep your upper arms stationary.
- Keep your wrists straight.
- Do not swing your arms.
- Squeeze through the backs of your arms at the top of each move.

Stand with your feet shoulder-distance apart, knees slightly bent. Lean forwards, keeping your abs contracted and back straight. Hold a dumbbell in each hand with your palms facing inwards. Lift your upper arms until they are parallel to the floor.

Extend the weights straight out behind you, without locking your joints. Hold for a split second and lower the weights back to the starting position.

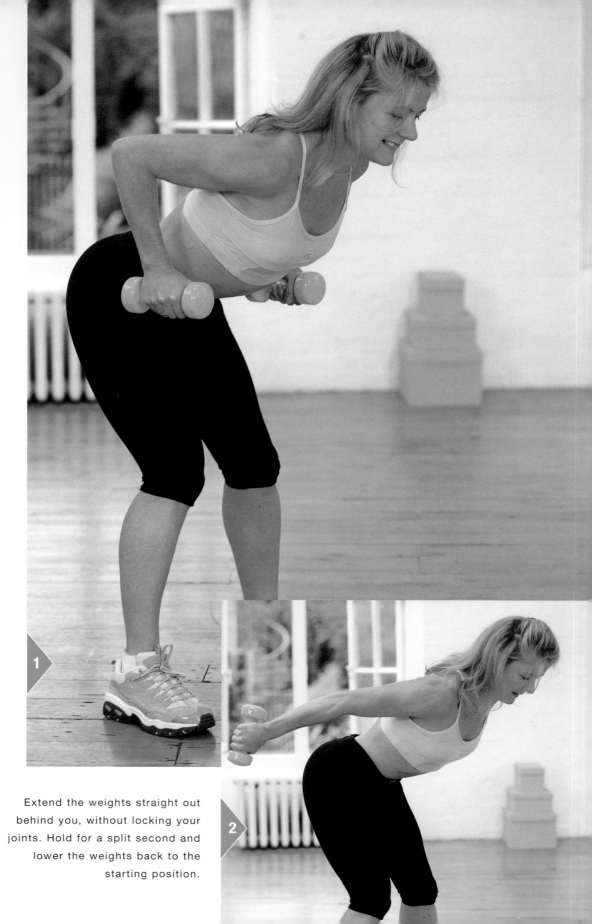

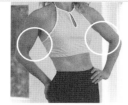

Biceps

Although we use this muscle group more frequently in everyday activities than the opposing tricep muscles, it is important to keep the biceps in shape. However, as women we are not as obsessed as Popeye was with this particular part of the anatomy. Filling the bicep muscles out will help tighten up any loose skin on the front of your arms. Concentration curls are one of the best exercises to help build definition in the muscle because they isolate the biceps. Choose one or two exercises and work your biceps twice a week.

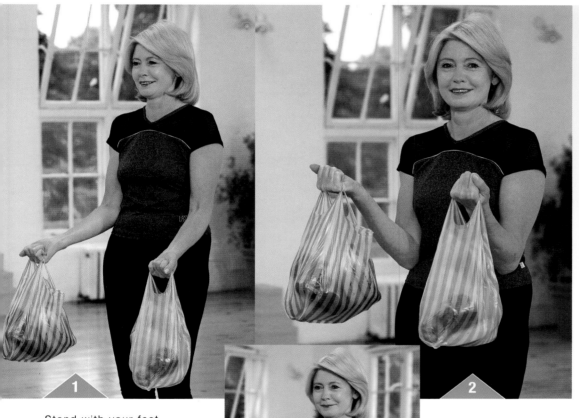

1 Stand with your feet shoulder-distance apart, knees soft. Hold a shopping bag or a dumbbell in each hand. Fully extend the arms without locking your elbow joint.

2 With your palms facing forwards, keep the wrists straight and lift the bags or dumbbells up to your shoulders, hold for a split second and release slowly.

Buy Your Biceps

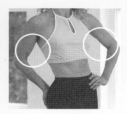

Equipment: 2–3kg weight or the equivalent in shopping bags 20 reps, 2 sets

If too much shopping is your excuse for not exercising then here is a perfect way to fit it in!

Watch Out!

- Keep your elbows snugly into your side throughout the exercise.
- Keep your wrists straight and in line with your forearm.

Band Biceps

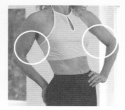

Equipment: a medium strength tubing band
20 reps, 2 sets

This versatile piece of tubing will shape up those arms anywhere and anytime.

Watch Out!

- Use control and not momentum with the band.
- Keep your wrists straight and elbows into your side.
- Your upper arm remains stationary.

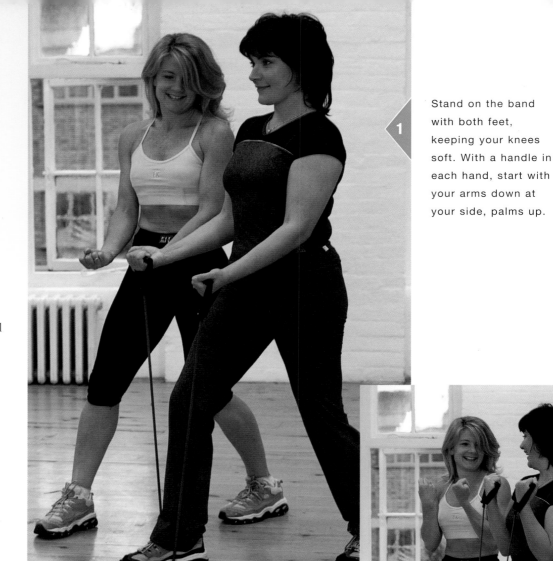

1 Stand on the band with both feet, keeping your knees soft. With a handle in each hand, start with your arms down at your side, palms up.

2 Keeping your wrists straight and elbows snugly into your side, pull both hands up to your shoulders and release slowly.

A Jenergy Challenge

Pull the band up and release slowly 10 times.
Pull the band up to your shoulders and release half way down instead of all the way down and repeat 10 times.
Now do single alternate curls with the band. Repeat 10 times on each side.

Sitting on a bench or chair, with a dumbbell in your right hand, place your right elbow on your right thigh. Fully extend your arm without locking your joint.

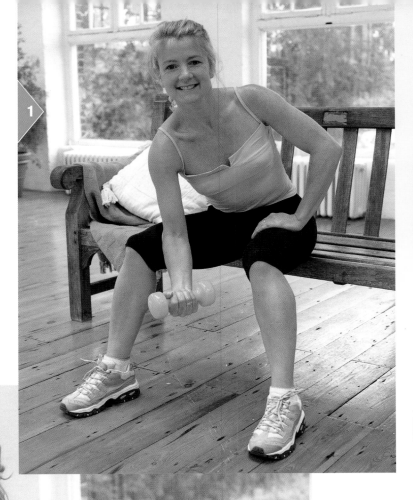

Concentration Curls

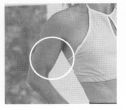

**Equipment: 2–5kg weight
12 reps, 2–3 sets**

This exercise has been hailed as one of the best for the biceps by top fitness trainers as it really isolates the muscle.

Watch Out!
- Keep your back straight.
- Do not allow momentum to lift the weight.
- Keep your wrist straight.

Keeping your wrist straight, pull the weight up to your shoulder. Hold for a split second and release slowly. Repeat on the other side.

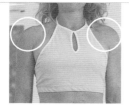

Shoulders

What a difference shapely shoulders can make to the whole shape of the body. Beautifully sculpted shoulders are truly an asset, and the next best thing to a Versace outfit on its hanger. Interestingly, the shoulder joint is the most mobile joint in the body, and quite susceptible to injury when overused.

In everyday life the posterior shoulder muscles are more neglected than the middle and front part of the shoulder, so it is vitally important that we take time to work them on a regular basis. Admittedly there is nothing worse than seeing fat accumulating around one's bra strap.

The rotator-cuff muscles, located in the shoulder, are a group of four, small muscles and have an equally important function. They act to rotate the arm medially and laterally and are vital for improving posture.

Work your shoulders two to three times a week and make sure you work the rear shoulder and the rotator-cuff muscles at least twice a week.

The Jenergy four part routine

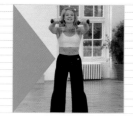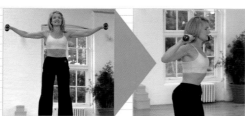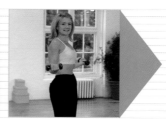

1. Front Raises

2. Lateral Raises

3. Overhead Press

4. Shoulder Rotations

When your shoulder strength has developed repeat the above four exercises in sequence with a 1kg weight placing extra effort on your technique. Do one set for each exercise.

Front Raises

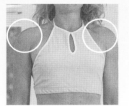

**Equipment: 1–2kg weight
8–10 reps, 2 sets**

This particular exercise will work the front part of the shoulders, giving them strength and lean definition.

Watch Out!

- Do not lock your elbows.
- As you lift, lengthen the weights away from your body.

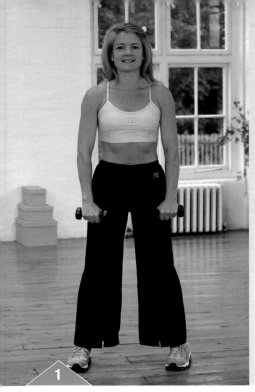

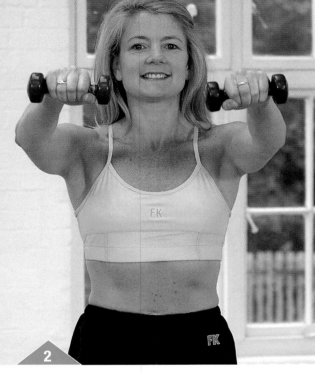

1 Stand with your feet slightly apart, knees soft and abs contracted. Start with the weights down in front of you, palms facing down.

2 Keeping your elbows slightly bent, lift the weights up to shoulder level and lower slowly. Allow one count on the lift and two counts on the lowering.

Lateral Raises

**Equipment: 1–2kg weight
8–10 reps, 2 sets**

This exercise shapes up the middle part of the shoulders. Developing your shoulders gives more balance to your lower body.

Watch Out!

- Do not lock your elbows.
- Do not allow your shoulders to shrug up.
- Lengthen out by reaching away from your body.

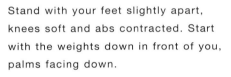

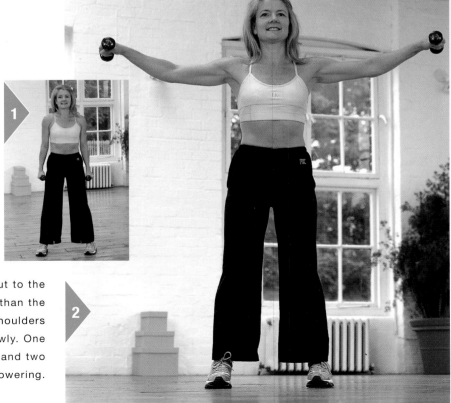

1 Stand with your feet slightly apart, knees soft and abs contracted. Start with the weights down by your side, palms facing inwards.

2 Lift the weights out to the side, no higher than the level of your shoulders and lower slowly. One count on the lift and two counts on the lowering.

Overhead Press

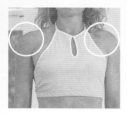

**Equipment: 1–2kg weight
8–10 reps, 2 sets**

Many women find this exercise difficult to perform. It is a good all-round shoulder exercise.

Watch Out!

- Use a push and pull principle and not momentum.

Extend the weights up and slightly to the diagonal. Pull them back until the weights are almost on your shoulders again.

Hold the weights just above your shoulders, palms facing forwards.

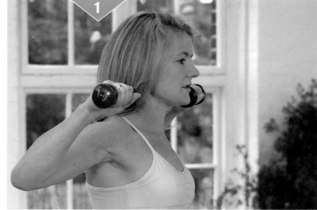

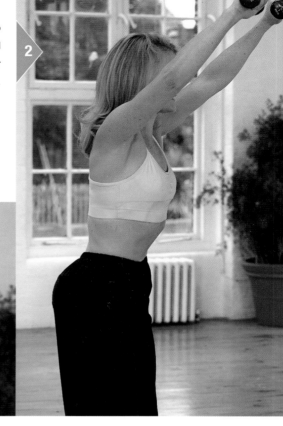

Shoulder Rotations

**Equipment: 1–2kg weight
8–10 reps, 2 sets**

This muscle is relatively weak in most women and this is not an exercise we tend to do in everyday activities. It is great for pulling those shoulders back and enhancing posture.

Watch Out!

- Keep your wrists straight.
- Keep your elbows into your sides.

Place your elbows into your side and lift your forearms until they are parallel to the floor. Palms up.

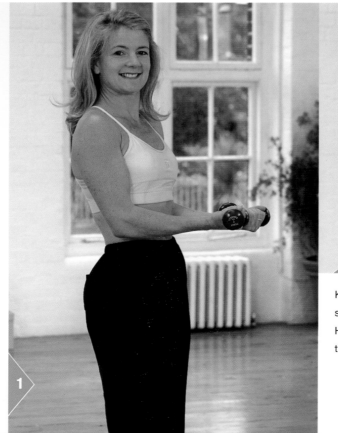

Keeping your elbows into your sides rotate the weights outwards. Hold for a split second and return to the starting position.

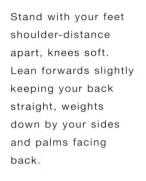

1 Stand with your feet shoulder-distance apart, knees soft. Lean forwards slightly keeping your back straight, weights down by your sides and palms facing back.

Rear Shoulder Raises

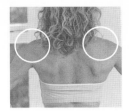

Equipment: 1–2kg weight
15 reps, 2 sets

Get rid of that bra-strap fat!

Watch Out!

- Do not hyperextend the neck.
- Keep your back straight.
- Lower your arms to your hips only.

Lift the weights straight behind you keeping your elbows soft. Hold for a split second and release slowly.

2

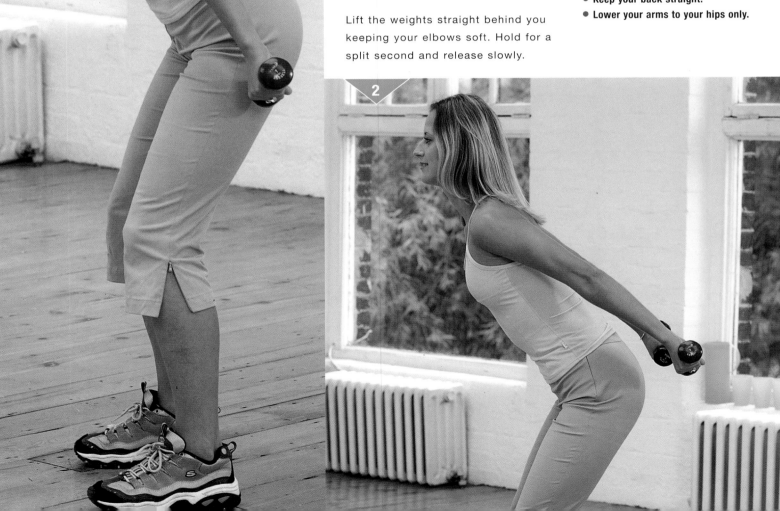

A BEAUTIFUL BACK

 **Perfect posture**

Sadly this part of our body tends to get neglected. Back pain is a serious problem and affects millions in the work place. Sitting all day long at a computer adds fuel to the fire as the muscles tend to passively slide away from the spine causing the shoulders to take on a rounded appearance.

However, many of us have simply shied away from taking a long look at the state of our bodies from behind. It's only when you spot yourself in the office party photos that you realise you should never have worn that backless dress. Having good muscle tone through the back is a beautiful asset. Once you have a strong toned back your whole body will take on a different appearance largely due to such an improvement in your posture. Besides, imagine never having to worry about that bra-strap fat again.

Smart tips for working your back muscles

- Work your upper-back muscles and stretch the chest muscles regularly, particularly if you sit at a computer all day. This will also lift and enhance the bust.
- Work your abdominals regularly to help support the spine.
- Work your lower-back muscles regularly.
- Stretch your hamstrings and hip flexors regularly as these muscles are closely associated with lower-back pain. (see Stretching p.102)

Do all of the back exercises at least twice a week.

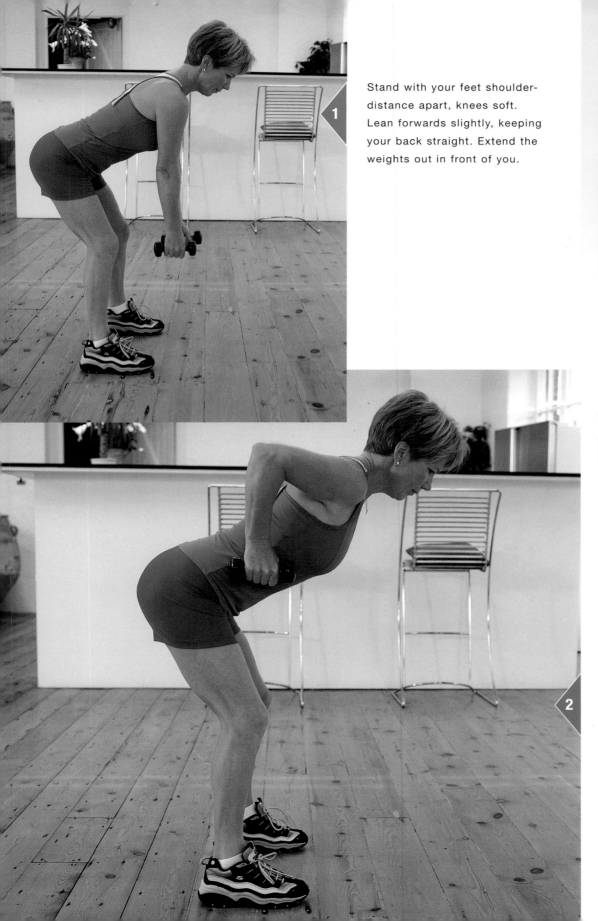

Stand with your feet shoulder-distance apart, knees soft. Lean forwards slightly, keeping your back straight. Extend the weights out in front of you.

Upper-back Strengthener

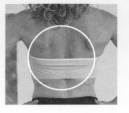

**Equipment: 1–3kg weight
12 reps, 2 sets**

This exercise tones the muscles across the middle and upper back. Imagine holding a marble between your shoulder blades to really feel the muscles working.

Watch Out!

- Do not let the shoulders shrug up – it's all back work.
- Keep your back straight.
- Do not hyperextend the neck.

Squeeze your shoulder blades together as you lift the weights up until your upper arms are parallel to the ceiling. Hold for a split second and release slowly.

Lucky Lats

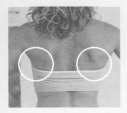

**Equipment: exercise ball
& 2–3kg weight
12 reps, 2 sets**

This muscle group is difficult to
work well without the use of
gym equipment. Fortunately, I
have one excellent exercise to
shape this part of the back. Use a
slightly heavier weight here for
maximum benefit.

Watch Out!

- Do not allow your back to arch.
  The rest of the body is not invited to
  the party.
- Fully extend the weight to feel the
  stretch through your lats.
- Do this exercise slowly.

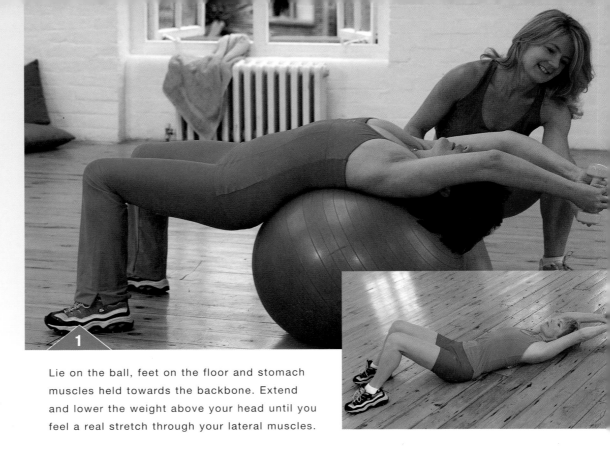

Lie on the ball, feet on the floor and stomach
muscles held towards the backbone. Extend
and lower the weight above your head until you
feel a real stretch through your lateral muscles.

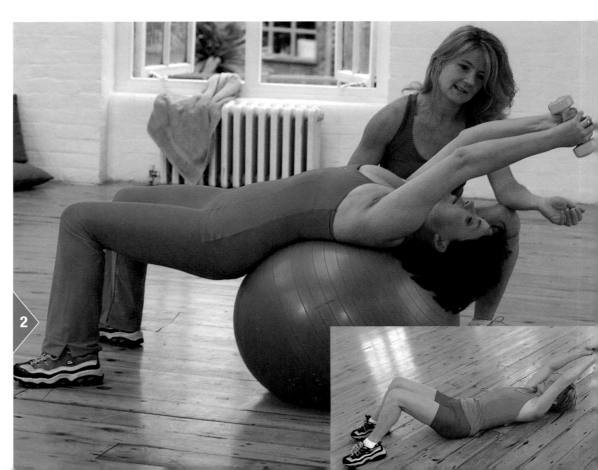

Keeping the elbows slightly bent,
lift the weight up to eye level and
release again making sure you
feel the stretch through the lats
each time you return.

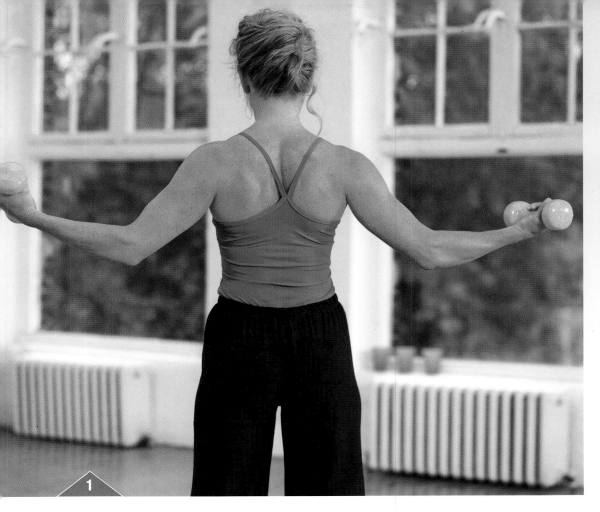

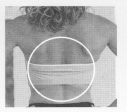

Super-shapely Back

Equipment: 1–kg weight
12 reps, 2 sets

This is one of my favourite back exercises. Technique here is vital, so really practise perfecting it.

Watch Out!

- Keep your shoulders relaxed – it is a back exercise.
- Squeeze your shoulder blades on the downward part of the movement.

1 Stand with feet shoulder-distance apart, knees soft and abs tight. Holding a dumbbell in each hand bring the elbows in and slightly behind your natural waistline.

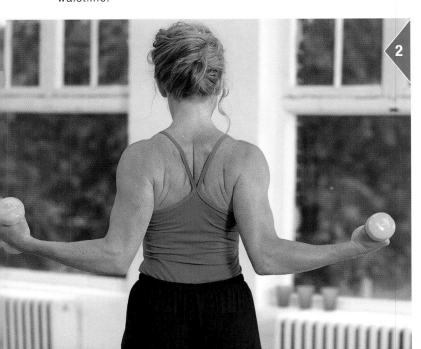

2 Extend the elbows out to 45° and as you bring them back into your side engage your back muscles first. Squeeze through your back muscles for a split second and go straight into the next repitition.

Lower-back Strengtheners

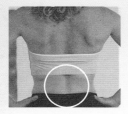

12 reps, 2 sets

Far too much focus is placed on working the abdominals alone, without working the lower back muscles. This can lead to injury, so make sure you work your lower back too.

Watch Out!

- Do not hyperextend the neck.
- Keep your chin towards your chest.

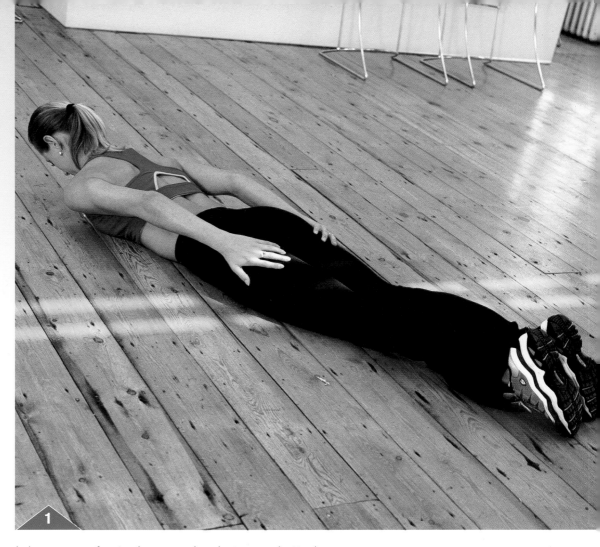

1

Lying on your front, place your hands on your buttocks.

A Jenergy Challenge

Try to do the lower-back strengtheners on the ball.

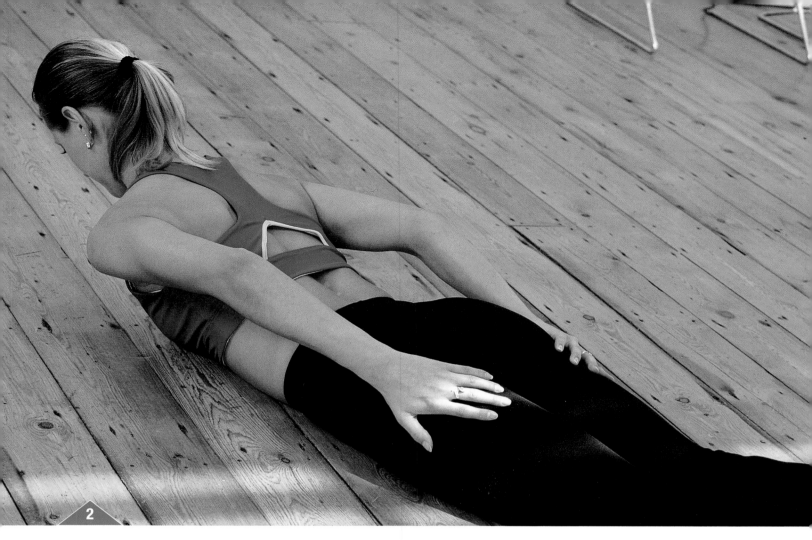

Keeping your chin towards your chest and feet firmly on the floor, lift the torso up, hold, and lower again.

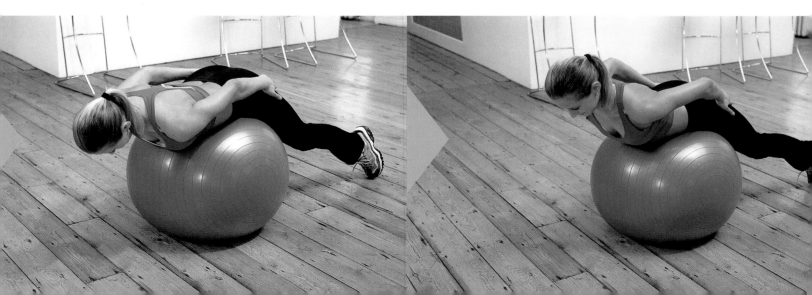

BUST FIRMERS

Very few women can perform twenty modified push-ups straight off. This exercise seems to frighten many women, perhaps because of its male orientation. With correct technique, twenty ladies' push-ups done three times per week will do wonders for developing firm, shapely arms and chest.

However, do not rely on this alone to develop your chest muscles. It is important to continue working your back muscles and stretching the chest muscles to improve posture and thereby enhance the chest. Work your chest muscles twice a week.

Ladies Push-ups

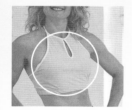

8 reps, 2 sets

You will be amazed, with a little persistence, how quickly the strength in your chest and upper body will develop.

Watch Out!

- Do not allow your back to arch and keep your abs contracted.
- Keep your head in line with your spine. There is a tendency to want to drop the head.
- Always check the positioning of your arms.

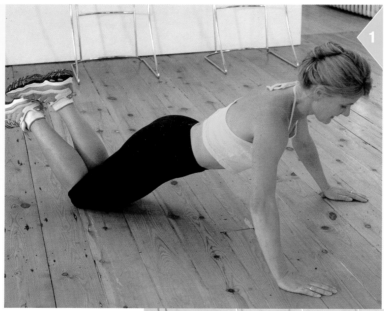

Come down onto your hands and knees. Cross your ankles and lift your feet up. Drop your hips until they are in line with your spine. Your arms should be a little further than shoulder-distance apart and in line with your face.

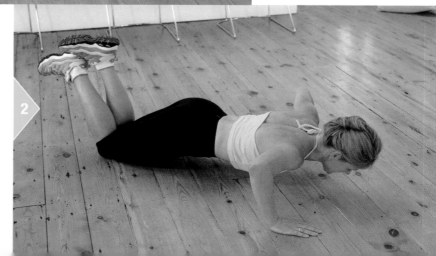

Exhale, and bend at your elbows lowering your body until your forehead just about touches the floor, and lift again.

Lying on an exercise ball or bench for height, make sure your head, neck and shoulders are supported. Keep your body supported by placing your feet under your knees and your back and abs strong. Hold a dumbbell in each hand. Start with your arms straight above you, palms facing in.

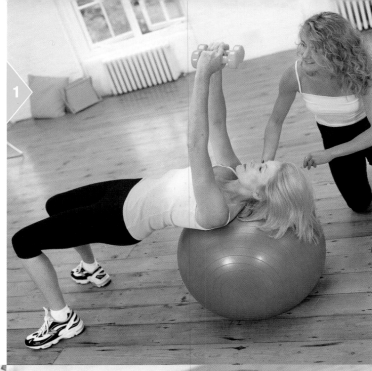

Chest Strengthener

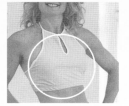

Equipment: exercise ball & 1–2kg weight
12 reps, 2 sets

A great alternative to push-ups and this exercise tends to isolate the chest muscles more.

Watch Out!

- Keep the rest of your body very stable.
- The movement comes through your shoulder joint.
- Keep your elbows locked into a slightly bent position.
- Squeeze your chest muscles on the upward part of the exercise.

Open your arms out until they are almost parallel to the floor. Bring your arms towards each other again, making sure you engage the chest muscles.

LOOK BEHIND

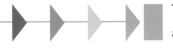

That lower-body solution! We sit on it all day and yet it causes us endless anguish. In a recent survey, a number of women were asked which body part they were most obsessed with getting into shape, the B word came out tops. When the same survey was aimed at men asking them which female body part they found most sexy when toned, guess what the answer was? Butts, bums, buns, buttocks!

The big picture should be evolving now as we start to pull everything together. We know that to change our body shape we need to train differently to the way we have in the past. We're going to learn how to perfect technique on each and every lower-body exercise. Once mastered, we can put the plan into action. The Jenergy training principles, which include high frequency, lower-body emphasis, core stabilisation and working with perfect technique should be implemented into each and every one of the lower-body exercises for maximum results.

The exercises challenge all the muscles through the lower body, often working more than one muscle group at a time. The kick-boxing and sports moves overload the buttock muscles, which will greatly improve the appearance of the bottom. You will gain strength and balance through the lower body with all the functional and standing-leg exercises. Then, to ensure not one muscle has been neglected, the floor work will isolate and tone specific muscles. Once you have altered the shape of your lower body by replacing unsightly dimpled fat for lean, sculpted and toned legs and buttocks, there will be a corresponding increase in your metabolism. With an increased RMR (resting metabolic rate) we burn more calories at rest.

Choose four to five exercises for each session and work your lower body four to six times a week.

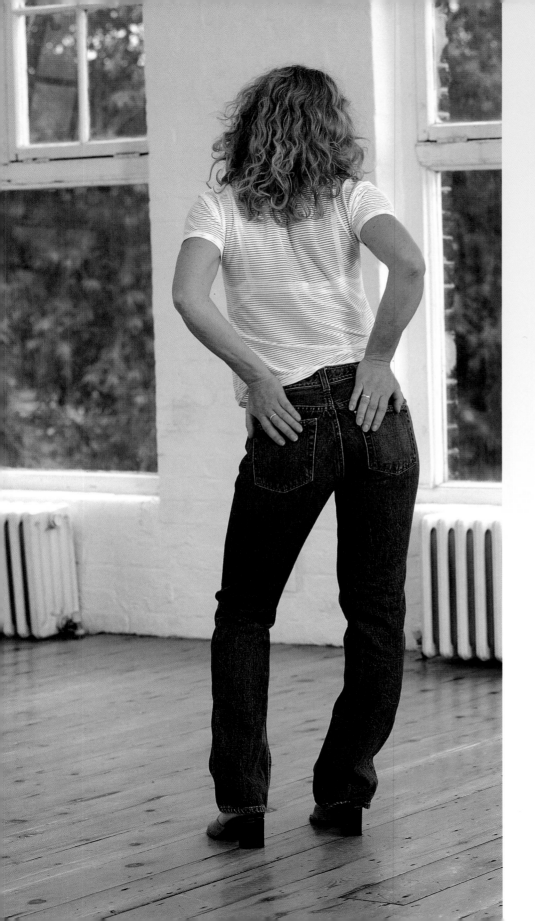

Smart tips for working that lower body

- If you are a beginner or have more than 15 pounds to lose start strengthening the muscles with the floor work exercises first. Doing too much standing-leg work can be stressful on the knees of beginners or overweight subjects.

- Squats and lunges are frequently used and are truly amazing at shaping the lower body provided they are done correctly. Most women do not know how to do a squat or lunge properly. Practise all these exercises until you have perfected them.

- Focus on using core stabilisation through all the standing-leg routines.

- Visualise keeping strong on the lifting phase and light on the lowering phase of all the standing-leg work.

Reverse Lunge

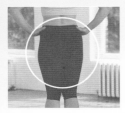

12 reps with each leg

It is quite easy to cheat with this exercise. Many women are afraid of engaging the muscles through the back leg to do the work, and end up with poor technique. To avoid this, practise reverse lunges to perfection before you take on too many reps.

Watch Out!

- Keep your upper body centred directly above both your legs.
- Make sure your pelvis is tilted to enable your body to push down and not forward (most common mistake).
- Make absolutely sure you have a right angle with your front knee.
- Remember to place more emphasis on the lifting than the lowering phase. You will recruit more muscle groups.

1 Feet together. Take a big step back with your left leg. As your left foot touches the floor lift the heel and tilt the pelvis forward. The back knee should be about 4 inches off the floor and the front knee should bend to no more than 90°.

2 Bring the left leg back up again and go straight into your next repetition.

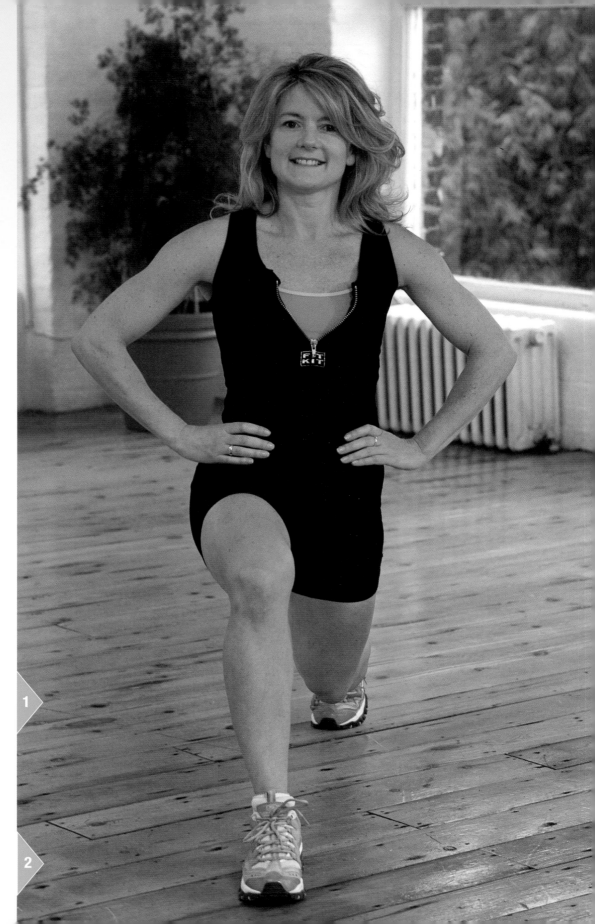

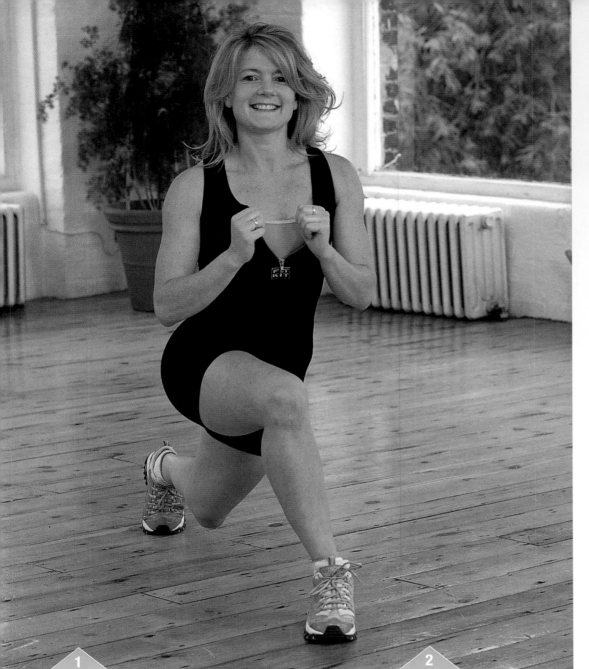

Crossover Reverse Lunge

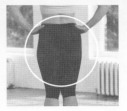

12 reps with each leg

This exercise is the same as the previous exercise with a slight crossover in the lunge which forces the inner thigh muscles to engage. One of the best all-round lower-body exercises. This is an advanced exercise, so plenty of practise makes perfect.

Watch Out!

- Keep a right angle with the front knee.
- Tilt the pelvis as you go into the lunge.
- Do not allow your back leg to cross over too much.
- Keep the knee and toe in line.

1 Feet together. Take a big step back and slightly across the centre of the body with your left leg. As your foot touches the floor lift your heel and tilt your pelvis forward.

2 Hold for a split second and bring your left leg back up again. Continue straight into your next repetition.

A Jenergy Challenge

Put the reverse lunge and crossover reverse lunge together. First on the left and then on the right leg.

Lunge for Lean and Lovely Legs

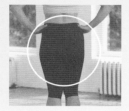

8 alternate lunges in one direction and 8 in the opposite direction

A 1999 study done at San Diego State University, involving 31 women aged 19–41, set out to find the most effective move for toning the buttocks. The walking lunge came second. Although it can be done anywhere, anytime and only takes minutes to do, this exercise looks deceptively simple and therefore should be started out slowly.

Watch Out!

- Keep a right angle with your front knee.
- Weight should be evenly balanced between both legs.
- Keep light on the downward part and strong on the lift.

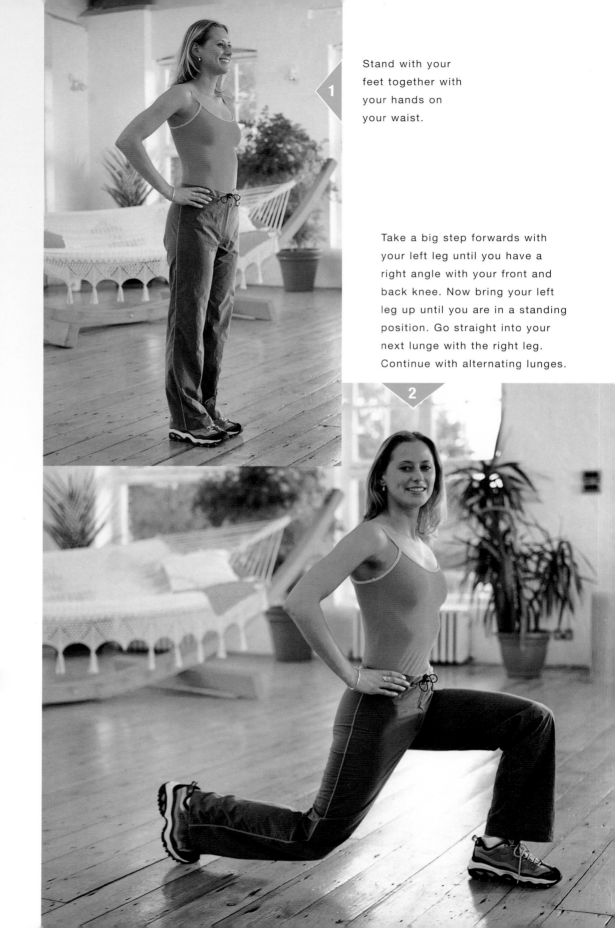

1 Stand with your feet together with your hands on your waist.

Take a big step forwards with your left leg until you have a right angle with your front and back knee. Now bring your left leg up until you are in a standing position. Go straight into your next lunge with the right leg. Continue with alternating lunges.

2

Start with feet shoulder-distance apart and both feet facing forwards with the left heel off the floor. Keeping the left heel lifted, squat to the left keeping your weight evenly distributed. Keep your back straight and push your hips out behind you.

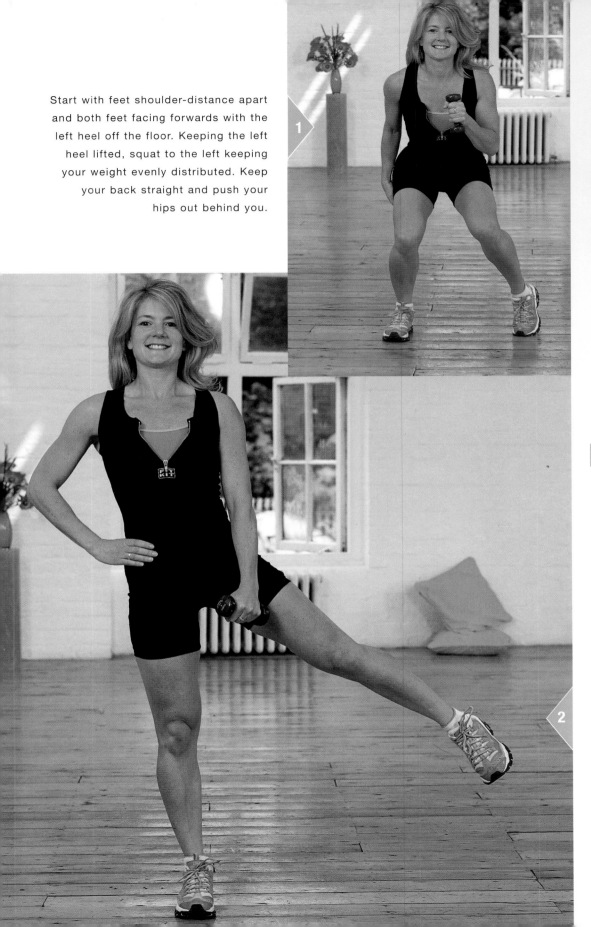

Squat and Tone with Triceps Extension

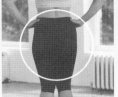

**Equipment: 1kg weight
15 reps each side**

This is great for developing strength and balance through the lower body. The weight is optional if you want to work your triceps simultaneously.

Watch Out!

- Land softly and lift firmly. Imagine testing the water with your toe (soft down) and being pulled up by your hair (firm up).
- Keep both toes and knees facing forwards.
- Keep your torso vertical.
- Focus on core stabilisation.

Lift straight up again with force and extend the left leg out to the side (not too high). At this point hold and squeeze through the buttock and outer thigh muscles. Go straight into your next repetition.

Squat and Kick with Weight

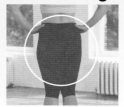

Equipment: optional 1kg weight
15 reps each side

This powerful exercise is a great challenge for the entire lower body and when teamed up with the squat and tone exercise, it works wonders.

Watch Out!

- Land softly and lift firmly.
- Keep both toes and knees facing forwards.
- When kicking, lift your knee first and then extend your foot. Do this movement with control.
- Focus on core stabilisation.

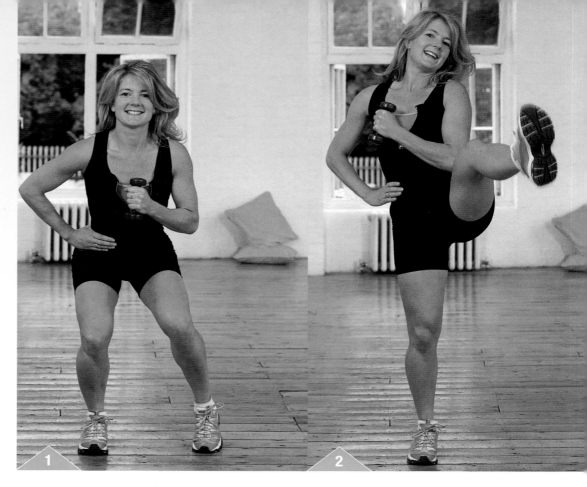

1

Start with feet shoulder-distance apart and both feet facing forwards with the left heel off the floor. Keeping the left heel lifted squat to the left keeping your weight evenly distributed. Keep your back straight and push your hips out behind you.

2

Lift straight up again and kick the left heel diagonally out in front of you. Land softly into your next repetition.

A Jenergy Challenge

Do the squat and tone and squat and kick exercises together. First on the left and then on the right.

 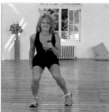 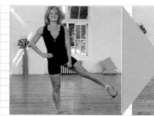 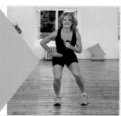 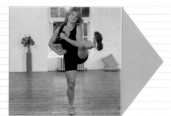

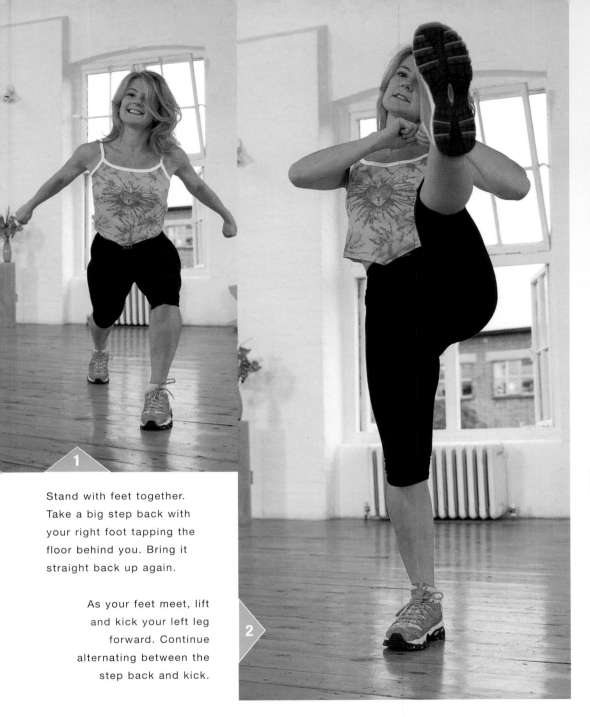

Kick Butt

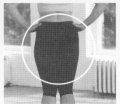

Repeat 12 reps on each side.

You can almost physically feel your muscles tighten up after doing this exercise. It targets almost every muscle in the lower body. Keeping the abdominals held towards the backbone makes it a great abdominal and back strengthener.

Watch Out!

- Your upper body is not invited to the party! Do not allow your torso to sway backwards or forwards.
- Focus on absolute torso stabilisation.
- Kick with control and do not throw the leg. Lift the knee first and then extend the foot.

1

Stand with feet together. Take a big step back with your right foot tapping the floor behind you. Bring it straight back up again.

2

As your feet meet, lift and kick your left leg forward. Continue alternating between the step back and kick.

A Jenergy Challenge

Step back once and kick 3 times. Repeat this routine 4 times on the right and 4 times on the left.

Outer-thigh Eraser

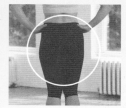

16 reps, 2 sets

Use a prop such as the back of a chair when you start out. Once you have developed strength and balance through the lower body try this routine without a prop. This is another leg exercise which requires extra effort – put something into this routine and you'll certainly reap the benefits.

Watch Out!

- Keep both knees soft.
- Keep your torso lengthened, abs tight and shoulders relaxed throughout the exercise.
- Keep your torso vertical.
- Squeeze your muscles on the downward part of the move.

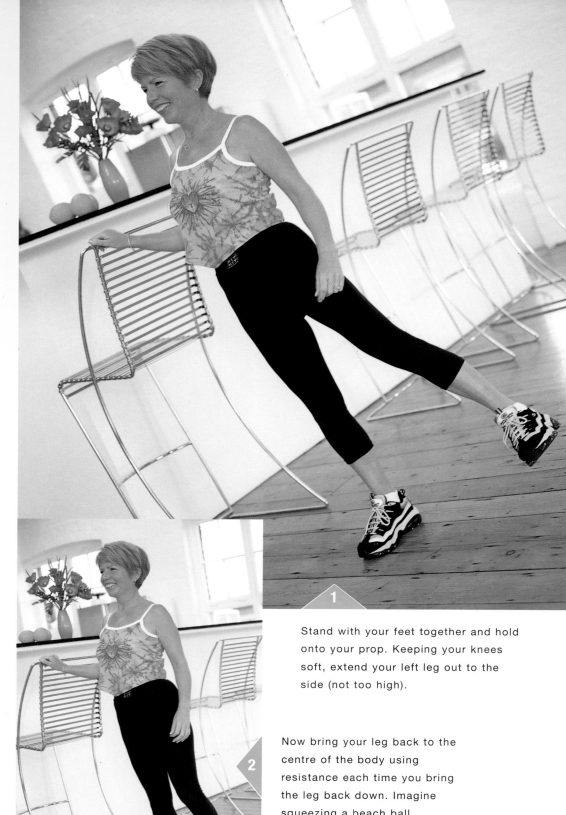

1

Stand with your feet together and hold onto your prop. Keeping your knees soft, extend your left leg out to the side (not too high).

2

Now bring your leg back to the centre of the body using resistance each time you bring the leg back down. Imagine squeezing a beach ball.

Place the band around your ankles (not too tight or loose). Stand with your feet shoulder-distance apart and knees and toes facing forwards.

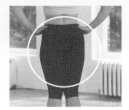

Alternate-leg Squats with Dynaband

**Equipment: medium band
16 reps each side**

A butt and thigh blaster which will rapidly trim and tone the lower body.

Watch Out!

- Do not let the band control you – make your muscles control the band.
- Keep knees, toes and torso facing forwards throughout.
- Focus on keeping the upper body stable – it is not invited to the party!
- Keep focus on torso stabilisation.
- Remember - only allow your foot to return half way back.

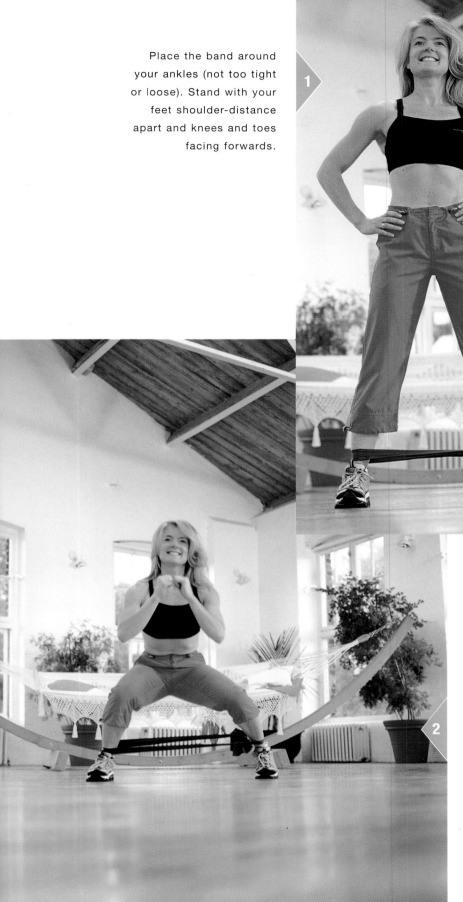

Squat to the right pushing your hips out behind you as you lower your buttocks. On the return only allow the foot to return half way back. Go straight into the left repetition.

Sport Buttocks

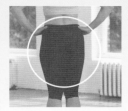

12 steps each side

Ever thought you had the fittest butt around and then went and played a game of squash and could hardly walk the next day? Not surprising, as this exercise works the butt the same way racket sports do – and more!

Watch Out!

- Do not allow your torso to sway back and forth. The movement comes through your hips and knees.
- Focus on torso stabilisation.
- Dip down into the move from the hips ensuring the knee does not go past a 90°.

1 Standing with both feet together. Take a big step forward with your left leg immediately followed by your right, keeping your back straight and lowering your body at your hips.

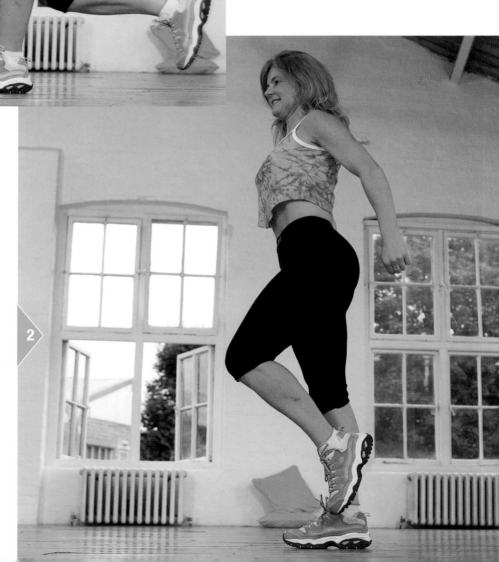

2 Step back with your right leg, followed by your left, back to the starting position. Continue your repetition. Visualise stepping low to hit that squash ball!

Stand on the edge of a step. Hold onto the banister for support. Move your right foot back until the ball of the foot is on the edge of the step. Hook your left foot around your right ankle.

Calf Raises

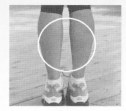

15 reps each side.

Did you know that shapely calves can be one of the most feminine parts of a woman's body? This exercise is sure to achieve just that.

Keeping your right knee soft, lift and slowly lower your right heel.

Watch Out!

- Lift and lower with control.
- Make sure your foot is facing forwards.
- Do not lock your knee joint when raising your heel.

LOWER BODY

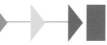

Lengthen and Strengthen

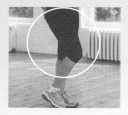

10–15 reps each side

This exercise really works on lengthening and strengthening the muscles throughout the entire leg.

Watch Out!

- Make sure your whole body is in a straight line.
- Do not lift your leg higher than 60°.
- Keep your abs contracted.
- Keep your breathing consistent.

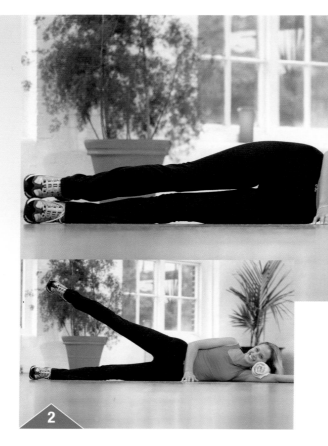

1

Lying on your side, place a cushion or rolled up towel between your head and shoulder. Straighten your body out by making sure your legs, hips and torso are all in one straight line. Imagine a giant ruler behind your body – make sure your body is pressed up against the ruler.

2

Without locking your knee joint lift and lower your top leg. As you lift your leg, lengthen it out and allow it to stretch away from your body, keeping the front thigh muscles contracted.

A Jenergy Challenge

Try adding 2 pulses between each rep.

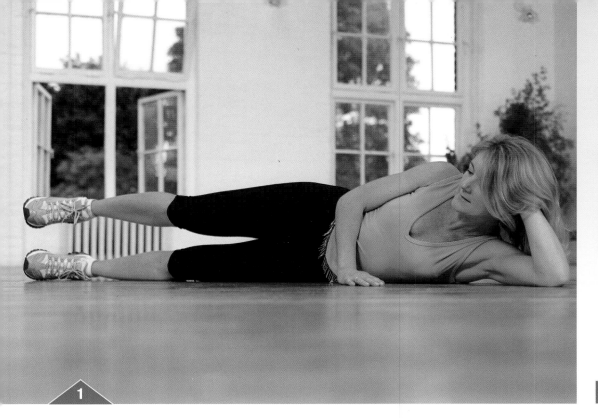

Hip and Thigh Toner

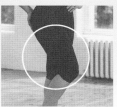

10–15 reps each side

An old favourite using the Jenergy technique to further challenge those hips and thighs.

1

Lying on your side place your head on your hand. With both legs slightly bent, keep the top hip forwards.

2

Lift your top leg to no higher than 60° and lower again. Work your muscles on the lowering phase by pushing through an imaginary resistance.

Watch Out!

- Do not allow your top hip to roll back.
- Keep both knees slightly bent.
- Do not lift your top leg higher than 60°.
- Focus on resisting on the downward part of the exercise.
- Keep your abs contracted.

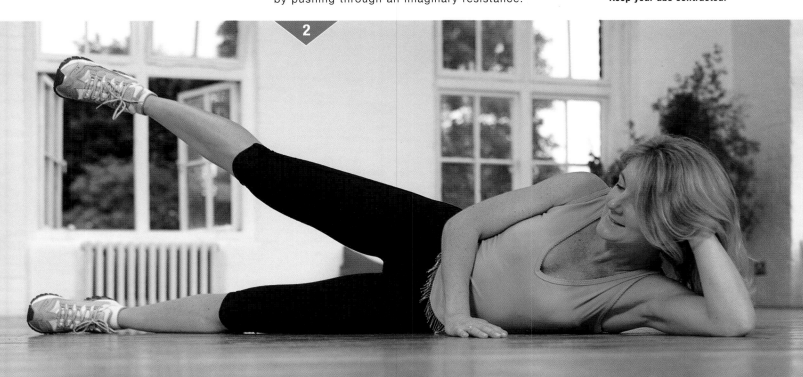

Hip and Thigh Ultra-toner

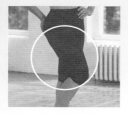

10–15 reps each side

A time-efficient exercise which, when done correctly, targets the hips, thighs and buttocks.

Watch Out!

- Do not allow your top hip to roll back, especially on the outward rotation.
- Keep both knees slightly bent.
- Resist on downward part of the exercise.

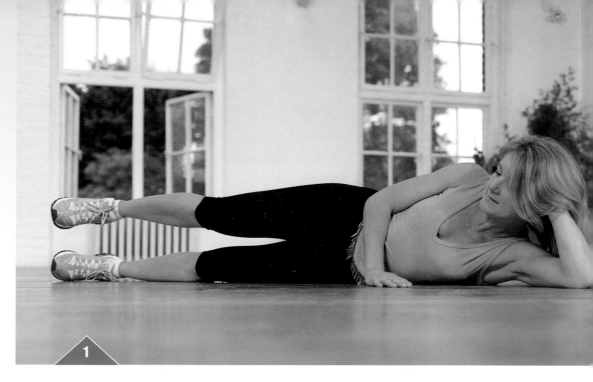

1

Assume the same position as the previous exercise.

Lift your top leg to no higher than 60°, and then without letting your hips roll back, rotate your leg outwards squeezing through your buttocks. Then, rotate your leg inwards and lower again with resistance. Continue with your reps.

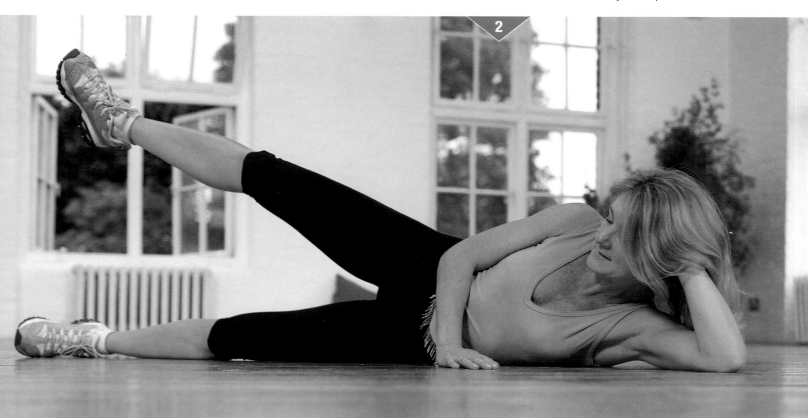

2

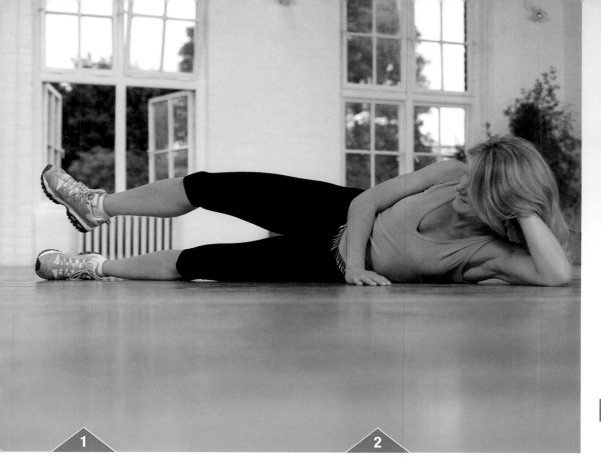

1

2

Diamond Legs

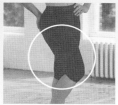

10–15 reps each side

Diamonds are a girl's best friend – this exercise will become your best friend when you see how it shapes up those buttocks and legs.

Watch Out!

- Keep your hips forward
- Keep a diamond shape between your legs.
- Squeeze through your muscles as you lower your leg.
- Keep your abs contracted.

Following on from the previous exercise, hold the top leg in the outward rotation position (without letting the hips roll back).

Keeping a diamond shape between your legs, pull your top heel towards your bottom heel, so once again the resistance is on the downward part of the exercise. Lift your leg again and continue with your reps.

A Jenergy Challenge

Perform the previous three exercises in sequence. First on your right leg and then on your left.

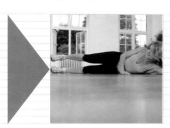
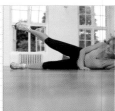
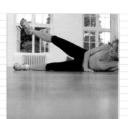
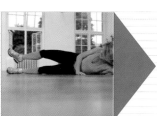

Knee to Floor and Extend

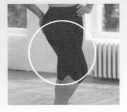

10–15 reps each side

A quick, effective exercise to complete that lower-body toning.

Watch Out!

- Do not throw your top leg. It is a push and pull movement.
- Make sure your knee comes all the way to the floor and your leg fully extends.
- Keep your hips forward and your abs contracted.

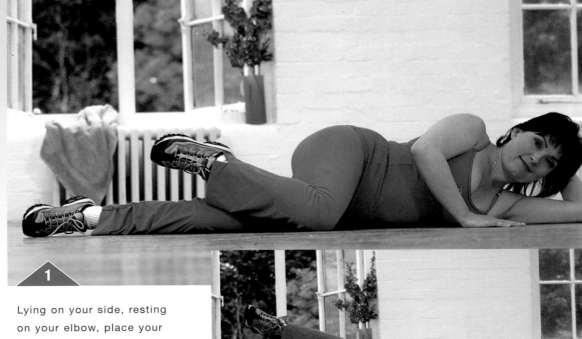

Lying on your side, resting on your elbow, place your top knee on the floor in front of you.

Extend your top leg out and up in front of you. Return to the start position and continue with your reps.

Deep External Rotators

10 reps each side

This exercise really gets into the deepest layers of the buttocks giving them that pert shape we all dream of.

Watch Out!

- As you rotate your top knee outwards really squeeze through your buttocks.
- Do not allow your top hip to roll back

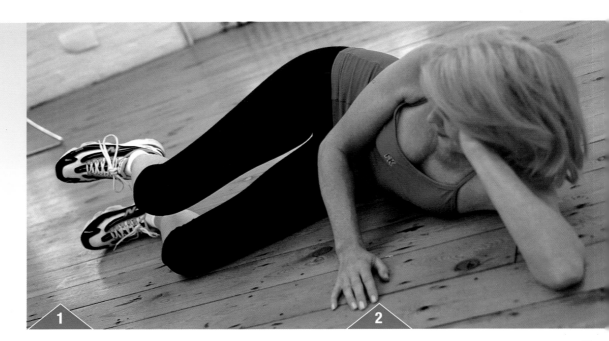

Lying on your side, resting on your elbow, bring both knees to a right angle in front of you. Lift your top leg about 2 inches from the bottom leg.

Now rotate the top knee a few inches further keeping your hips forward and return.

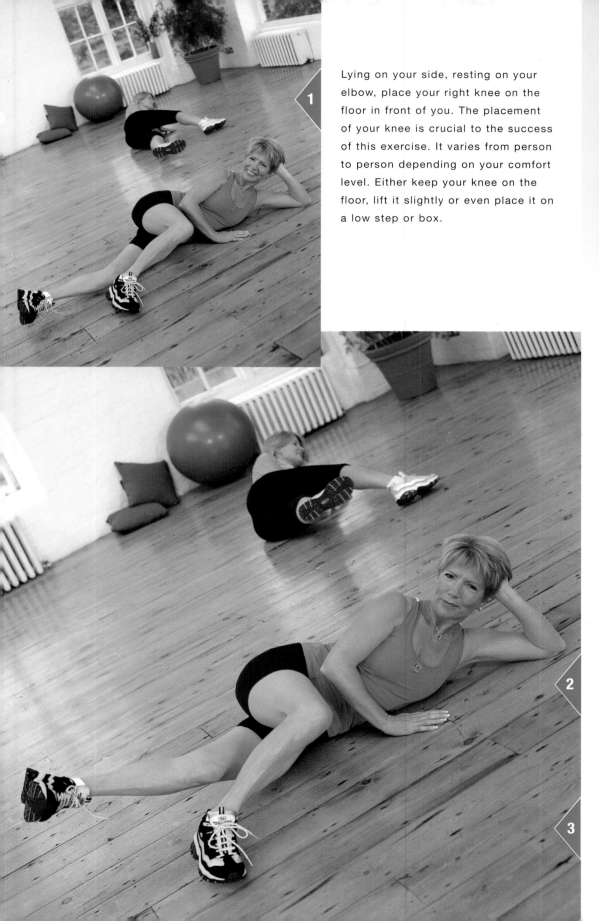

Lying on your side, resting on your elbow, place your right knee on the floor in front of you. The placement of your knee is crucial to the success of this exercise. It varies from person to person depending on your comfort level. Either keep your knee on the floor, lift it slightly or even place it on a low step or box.

Inner-thigh Raises, Pulses and Circles

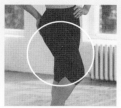

12 reps in each direction

The following leg routine is superb at shaping up the inner thighs, if done with the correct body alignment.

Watch Out!

- The underneath leg should be in front of the level of your hips. This is very important! If not it can pull on your lower-back muscles.
- Do not lock the knee of your exercising leg.
- Keep your foot in a slightly flexed position.

Keeping your left knee slightly bent, lift your left leg with force, hold it for a split second and lower again, for 12 reps. Now hold your leg at the top of the move and pulse, with control, for 8 reps.

Now circle the leg 8 times in one direction and 8 times in the other direction. Repeat on the other side

Cellulite-free Hamstrings and Buttocks

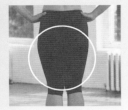

12 reps each side

This is the best exercise to shape up the back of the thighs. These are the most untoned muscles on a woman's body and can take on that unsightly orange peel look. They are relatively weak in most women compared to the opposing front thigh muscles which we tend to use more in everyday activities. Do this exercise at least twice a week.

Watch Out!

- Keep your lower back pressed to the floor by keeping the pelvis tilted throughout the exercise.
- Keep your knees together.
- Keep your weight evenly balanced and do not tilt your pelvis to either side.

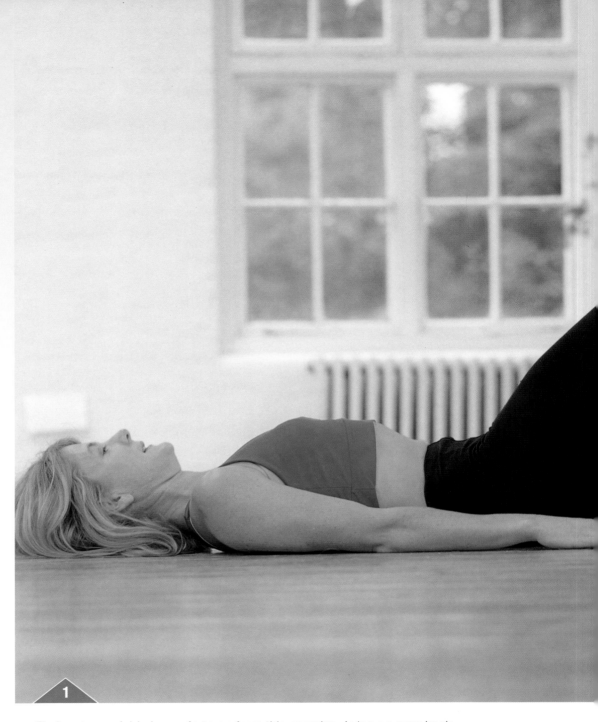

1

Find a step or fairly low sofa to perform this exercise. Lying on your back place your left foot on the end of the hard surface you are using and shift your buttocks about 2 feet away. Keep your buttocks on the floor and line your right leg up with your left knee keeping the right knee slightly bent.

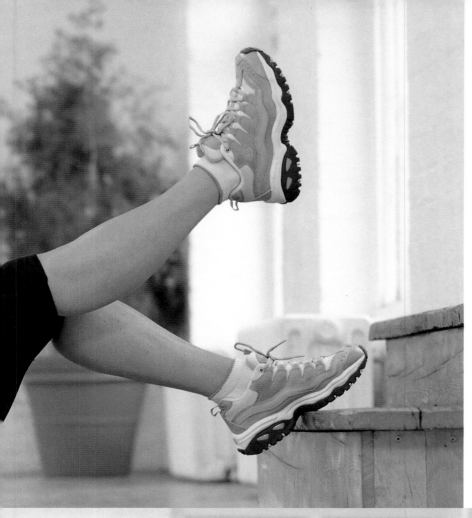

Keeping your knees locked together,
lift the buttocks off the floor, hold for a
split second and lower again.

2

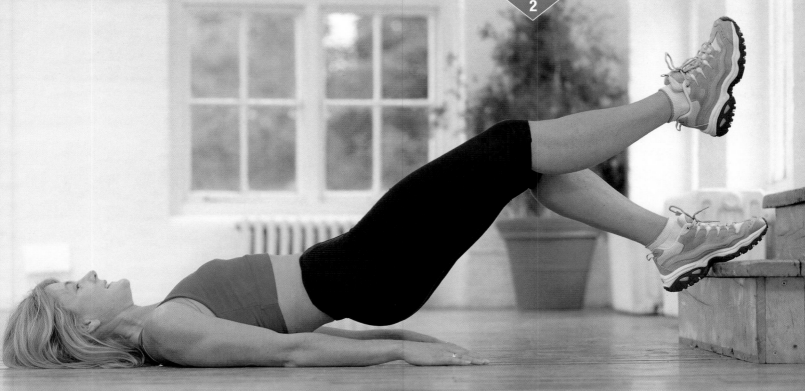

FAB ABS FOREVER

This muscle group seems to be the most talked about and yet the least understood of all the muscle groups. To find out how technically minded a client is, I normally get them to perform the stomach crunch. The way they do this exercise gives me an immediate understanding on their technical ability. It is surprising how few people really understand the way to work their abdominals properly.

Peter Fransis, director of the Biomechanics Laboratory at San Diego State University, explains that the key to a flat stomach is knowing which muscles to isolate. Poor technique won't work your abdominals as well. According to Fransis, women trying to obtain a six-pack face several obstacles. We tend to store fat below and around the belt. 'You can have strong abdominal muscles and a low percentage of overall body fat and still have a layer of fat there,' he says.

The abdominals are composed of four different muscles that work cooperatively, so if you want to see results, you have to strengthen all four muscles together. Many exercise classes place too much emphasis on the rectus abdominal with little focus placed on the all important oblique and transverse muscles. In addition, many abdominal exercises are difficult to perform properly and for this reason many women fail to achieve a flat stomach.

Understanding the four abdominal muscle groups is crucial to the success of your abdominals project. As mentioned previously, the abdominals work to stabilise and move the body. So, whilst it is important to do isolation work which strengthens all four muscles, it is equally important to continue using them in everyday activities such as walking, sitting and standing. In fact, by doing this half the battle is won when it comes to keeping your stomach muscles in shape. 'Keep those abs zipped up' is one of my favourite sayings. Do not expect a flat stomach on doing the abdominal exercises alone. Include cardiovascular exercise to help burn fat and eat sensibly. To ensure proper muscle balance make sure you work your back muscles regularly.

Work your abdominals three times a week, choosing two to three exercises which incorporate the rectus and oblique muscles.

The abdominal muscles

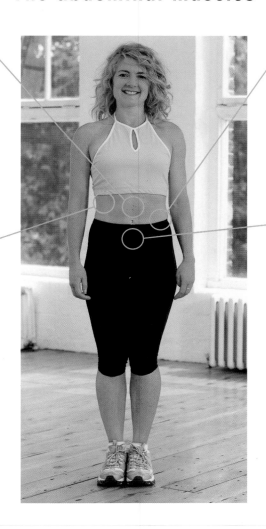

Rectus abdominal

The largest muscle of the group. This muscle runs continuously from the rib cage to the pubis. It enables you to bend at the waist. There are no upper and lower abs as many people believe.

External obliques

The outermost layer of muscle which runs diagonally down your sides. An easy way to remember the orientation of this muscle is to picture these fibres forming a V-shape.

Internal obliques

Right beneath the external obliques lie the internal obliques. These muscles allow you to twist and bend to the side. Picture these fibres forming an inverted V-shape.

Transverse abdominal

The deepest muscular layer in the abdominal wall. The fibres of this thin muscle run horizontally, encircling the abdominal cavity. These muscles are used when you cough or exhale forcefully. They contract when the other three are working but can't be worked in isolation.

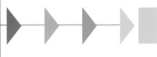

Pelvic Floor

Many of you were probably brainwashed with this exercise during pregnancy and yet so many women tend to neglect it a few months after giving birth. This is unfortunate as it is crucial to the success of flat, firm abdominals. The firm, supportive pelvic floor muscles help to hold the bladder, womb and bowel in place.

Pelvic floor muscles can become weak and sag because of childbirth, lack of exercise, the change of life, or just getting older. If you find you leak urine, especially with exercise or when you cough or sneeze, it is because the muscles have become weak and have less control.

By exercising the pelvic floor regularly the muscles will strengthen once again and will be able to give support. Like any other muscles in the body, the more you exercise them, the stronger they will be. An added bonus is that once these muscles are firmed up, your sex life will improve dramatically.

How to do pelvic floor exercises properly

Sit comfortably with your knees slightly apart. Imagine you are sitting on the toilet and passing urine. Without moving your buttocks and legs, imagine trying to cut off the urine flow. Really pull up from underneath and be aware of the skin around the back and front passage tightening and being pulled up and away from the chair. You can occasionally try the 'stop test' when emptying your bladder. Stop the flow about half way through, relax again and empty the bladder completely. Do not get into the habit of doing this test every time you pass urine. Only practice once a day at the most. You can try doing this exercise when driving, standing at the checkout till or just sitting watching TV.

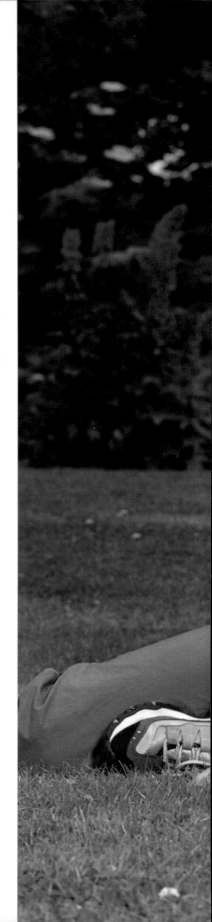

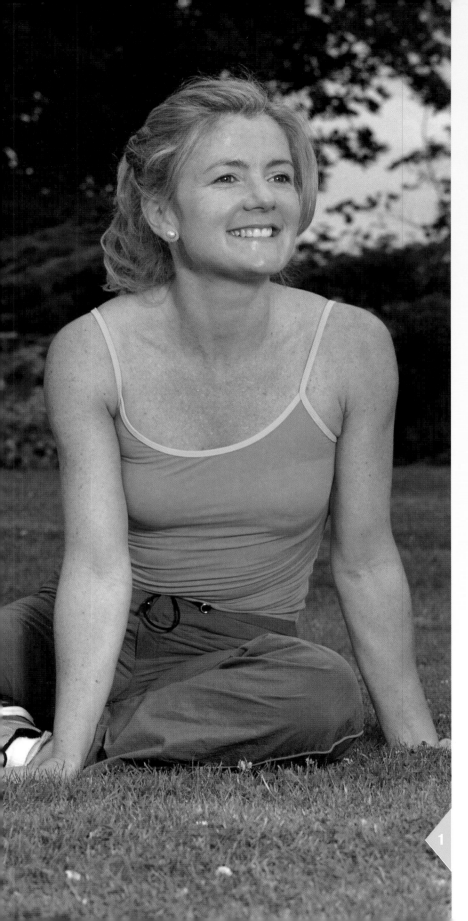

Smart tips for svelte abs

- Always keep the abs held towards the backbone and do not allow them to pop out.

- No other body part is invited to the party! When working the abdominals keep the lower body stabilised.

- Avoid using the neck and shoulders! Always keep an imaginary apple between your chin and chest to prevent you from getting neck strain.

- Do not allow the shoulders to shrug up. When lifting from the torso, keep the shoulders relaxed by bringing the elbows in slightly.

- Control not momentum! On each and every rep come up with relative force, hold for a split second and lower slowly.

- Breath correctly. Exhale on the lift or contraction.

- When doing a stomach crunch collapse the breastbone towards the naval in a rolling fashion and do not try and lift the torso upwards.

1

Be sure to work those pelvic floor muscles anytime, anywhere.

The Stomach Crunch

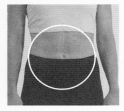

12 reps, 2 sets

This works the rectus abdominal. If you are only feeling it through the top part of the abdominals, don't worry. This means you are lifting through the top of the body. As your abdominals gain strength you will be able to identify with the full length of the muscle.

This is one of the most popular abdominal exercises, but studies have proved it is not the most effective. The reason being is that it activates the hip flexors, encouraging them to work more and the abdominals less. However, this particular crunch works wonders because the position of the legs deactivates the hip flexors, forcing the abdominals to do the work.

Watch Out!

- Keep an imaginary apple between your chin and chest.
- Relax your shoulders by keeping your elbows in slightly.
- Keep your abs contracted.
- Exhale on the contraction.

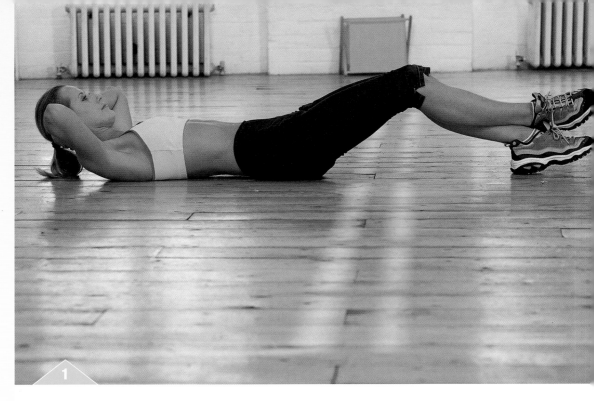

1 Lie on your back, knees together, ankles crossed and toes up. Place your hands behind your head and lift the head and shoulders slightly off the floor into the starting position.

Now lift a further 2–4 inches drawing the breastbone towards the navel. Hold for a split second and lower slowly.

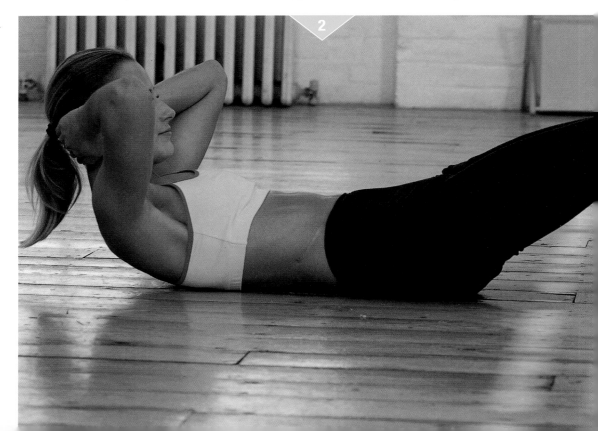

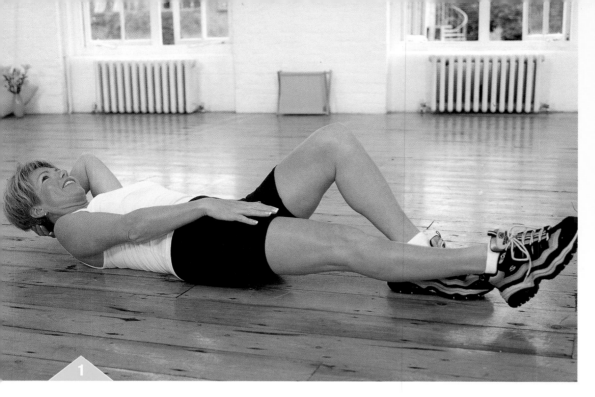

Extended-leg Reaches

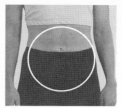

15 reps each side

This exercise works the rectus abdominal. The oblique muscles engage here too and sometimes this can be felt through the middle of the back. Don't mistake this for back pain. However, do this exercise with caution and always listen to your body.

Watch Out!

- Keep the abs scooped towards the backbone.
- Keep that imaginary apple between your chin and chest by looking at the foot of the extended leg.
- Make sure you lift straight up and do not allow your body to tilt to either side.

1

Lie on your back with your left knee bent. Extend your right leg out and hold it a few inches off the floor. Place your left hand behind your head and lift your head and shoulders just off the floor, placing the right hand on the right thigh.

Now lift a further 2–4 inches bringing the breastbone towards the navel. Hold for a split second and release.

2

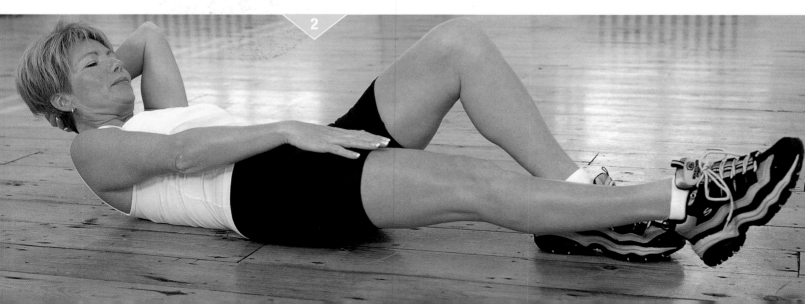

Crunch with the Ball

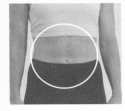

Equipment: 63cm ball
15 reps, 2 sets

This exercise works the rectus abdominal and the obliques. In a study done by Peter Fransis this exercise came out tops in order of effectiveness. Because you start with your back extended, this exercise forces your abdominals to work through a wider range of motion than most others. The obliques are also challenged by balancing your body on the ball.

Watch Out!

- Make sure your lower back is comfortably on the ball.
- Keep an imaginary apple between your chin and your chest.
- Relax your shoulders by bringing your elbows in slightly.

Lift your shoulders about 6 inches, drawing your breastbone towards your naval. Hold for a split second and lower again.

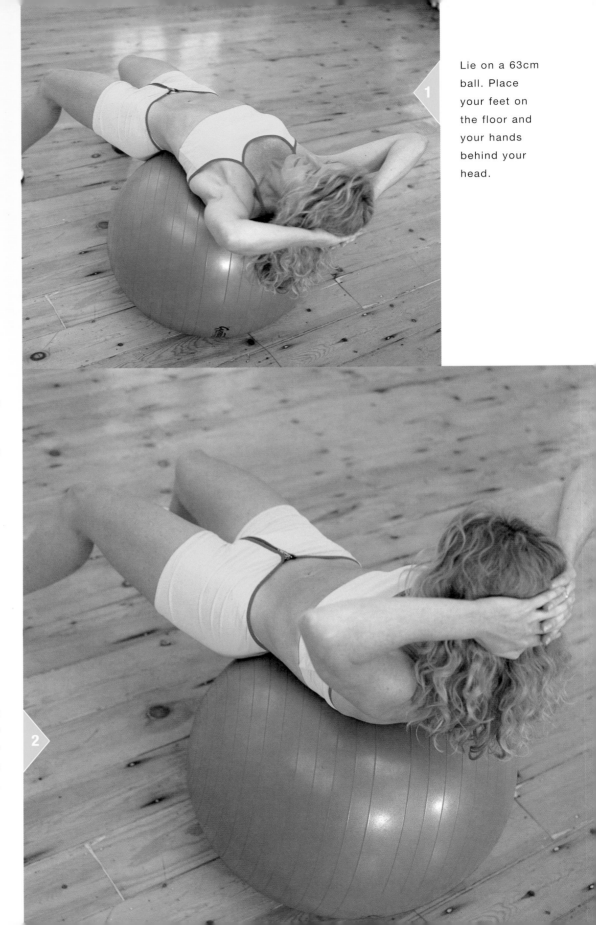

1 Lie on a 63cm ball. Place your feet on the floor and your hands behind your head.

2

Abs Towards the Backbone

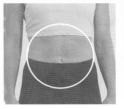

15 reps

This exercise works the obliques and transverse muscles. A great one for getting those abdominals back – especially good for back sufferers as the back muscles are not involved at all.

Watch Out!

- Only pull up on your abs. Do not alter the position of your back or tighten your buttocks.
- Breathe consistently throughout the exercise. Do not hold your breath.

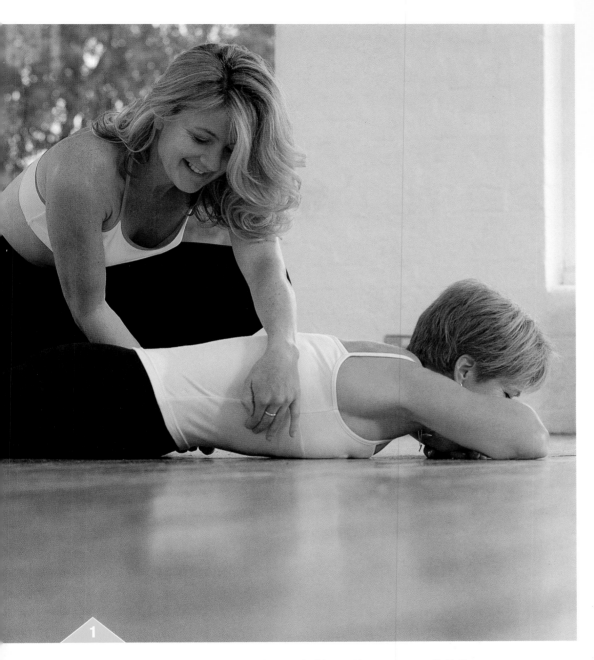

1

Lie flat on your stomach, legs together and chin resting on arms. Pull the lower part of your abs up towards the backbone. Hold for three counts and release for one. Imagine a golf ball being rolled underneath your abs.

Lift and Circle

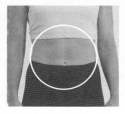

8 reps clockwise and 8 reps anti-clockwise

This exercise challenges all four abdominal muscles. A powerful stomach exercise.

Watch Out!

- Keep the circle narrow and do not sway too much to the left or right.
- Do not allow your abs to pop out. Keep them contracted.
- Avoid using your neck muscles by constantly being aware of that imaginary apple between your chin and chest.
- Keep your lower body stable. It is not invited to the party! Only the torso moves.

Now lift up towards the left and circle around to the right (clockwise), back to the start position. Repeat anti-clockwise changing your leg position.

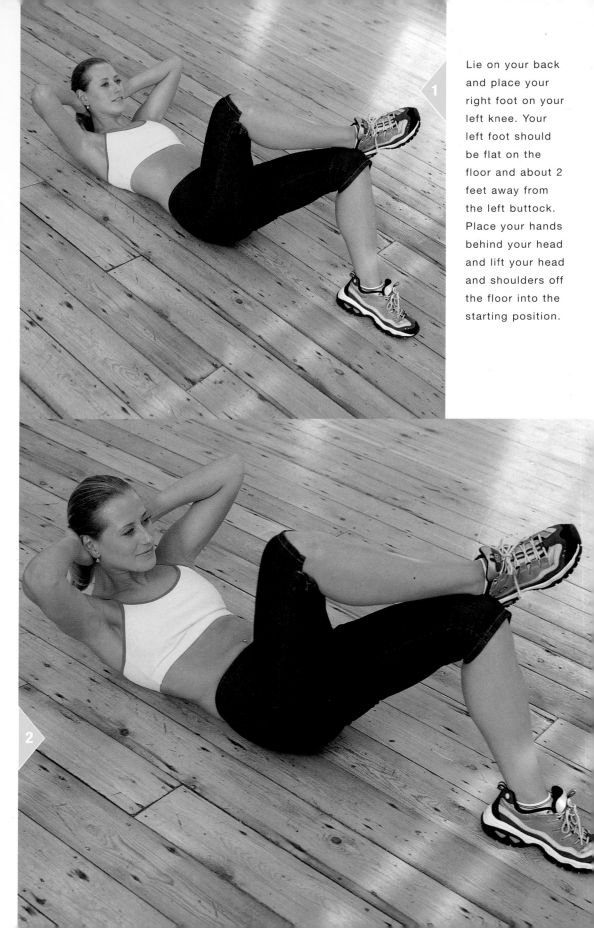

1 Lie on your back and place your right foot on your left knee. Your left foot should be flat on the floor and about 2 feet away from the left buttock. Place your hands behind your head and lift your head and shoulders off the floor into the starting position.

2

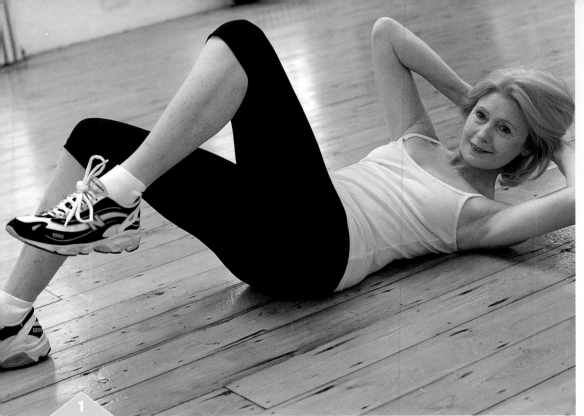

Waist Curl

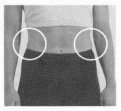

16 alternating each side

This exercise works the external and internal obliques.

Watch Out!

- Keep that imaginary apple between your chin and chest by keeping your head in the same position throughout.
- When curling across, aim your nose towards the outer thigh.
- Keep your head and shoulders off the floor until the exercise is complete.

Lie on your back, knees bent, feet on the floor, hands behind your head with your elbows in slightly. Curl your torso up and bring your right elbow to your left knee. Hold and lower without putting your shoulders back on the floor. Repeat on the other side.

Lie on your back, knees up and feet flat. Place your left hand behind your head and your right hand on your right outer thigh. Lift your head and shoulders up a few inches into your starting position.

Now lift and aim your left armpit towards your right knee by drawing the rib cage towards your naval. Hold, and release to the starting position.

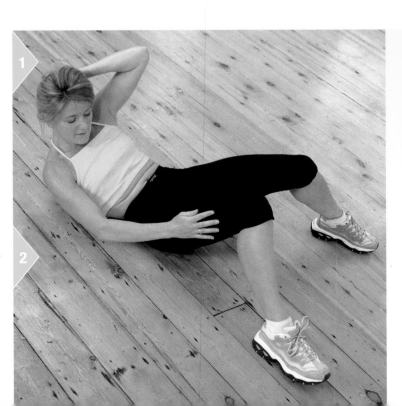

Waist Away

15 reps each side

This exercise works the external and internal obliques. Such a simple technique. If you really implement that split second, it will work wonders on your waistline.

Watch Out!

- Use control here. Lift with force, hold at the top of the move and lower slowly.
- Aim your armpit towards the knee. Do not go too far across.
- Keep your shoulders relaxed and your abs contracted.

Bridge

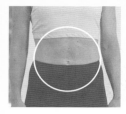

5 reps

The obliques work very hard here to stabilise the body. The transverse muscles are challenged too.

Watch Out!

- Make sure you keep your back absolutely straight and do not hyper-extend your neck.
- When leaving the position place your knees on the floor first to avoid any unnecessary strain on your back.
- Breathe consistently throughout the exercise.

A Jenergy Challenge

Try the exercise with the ball when you have built up your ab muscles.

Start in the push-up position but with weight resting on forearms. Keeping your back straight and head in line with the spine, contract your abs up to your backbone and hold for 8–10 seconds. Rest briefly before repeating.

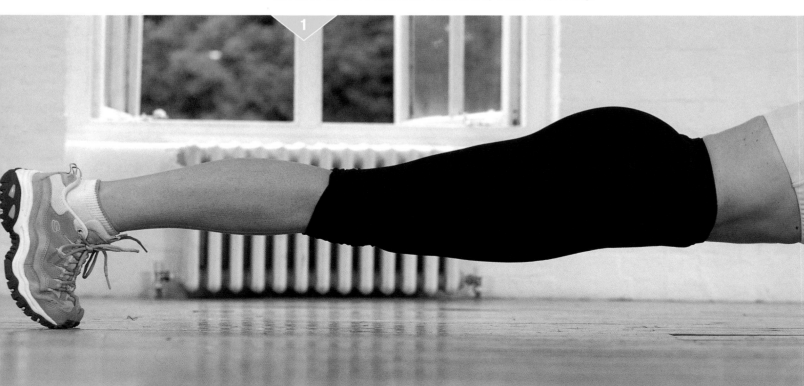

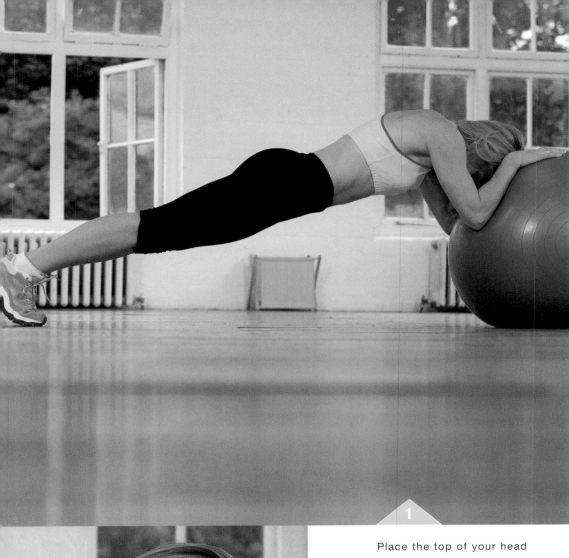

With the Ball

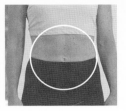

**Equipment: 63cm ball
5 reps**

This is far more challenging on the obliques as you have to keep the ball steady. Only do this exercise when you have built strength through the abdominal muscles and can master the bridge exercise with ease.

Watch Out!

- Make sure you keep your back absolutely straight and do not hyper-extend your neck.
- When leaving the position place your knees on the floor first to avoid any unnecessary strain on the back.
- Breathe consistently throughout the exercise.

1

Place the top of your head and the elbows on a 63cm ball. Lengthen the body out until it is straight. Contract the abs towards the backbone and hold for 8–10 seconds. Rest briefly before repeating.

STRETCHING

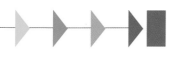

We've been told it's good for us to spend more time stretching at the end of every workout. It relieves stress and lengthens the muscles. But, as we extend our leg towards the ceiling to 'feel that stretch', how many of us understand exactly what we are trying to achieve?

Interestingly, stretching is something we do unconsciously in everyday activities. Take the morning stretch when you get out of bed. You don't jump up and sprint to the bathroom. If you have been sleeping in a certain position for a while you stretch and try to limber up. Even dogs and cats have a good old stretch upon awakening. Why, then, after working out are we so eager to finish up, look at our watch and go. Part of the reason is that many of us don't understand the tremendous benefits of stretching and we tend to place more emphasis on cardiovascular and strengthening. In addition, being inflexible makes us more likely to ignore the problem rather than tackle it.

Becoming flexible will open a whole new dimension to your fitness goals. Recent studies suggest that it is vital to include flexibility training in all fitness programmes, supporting evidence that injuries do occur as a result of tight or stiff muscles. Most professionals agree that static stretching is the safest way to develop flexibility. Ballistic (bouncing) stretching is not recommended and can indeed cause injury. Hold each stretch for at least 20 seconds. Breathe deeply and consistently into each stretch. When you feel you are at your furthest point, breathe deeply and try to increase the stretch a little further, without feeling any discomfort.

Finally, to achieve a fantastic overall look after working so hard at tightening and toning the muscles you need to have good flexibility. Shortening the muscles during strength training exercise will certainly tone them up. Lengthening them with flexibility exercises will make all the difference to the finished look.

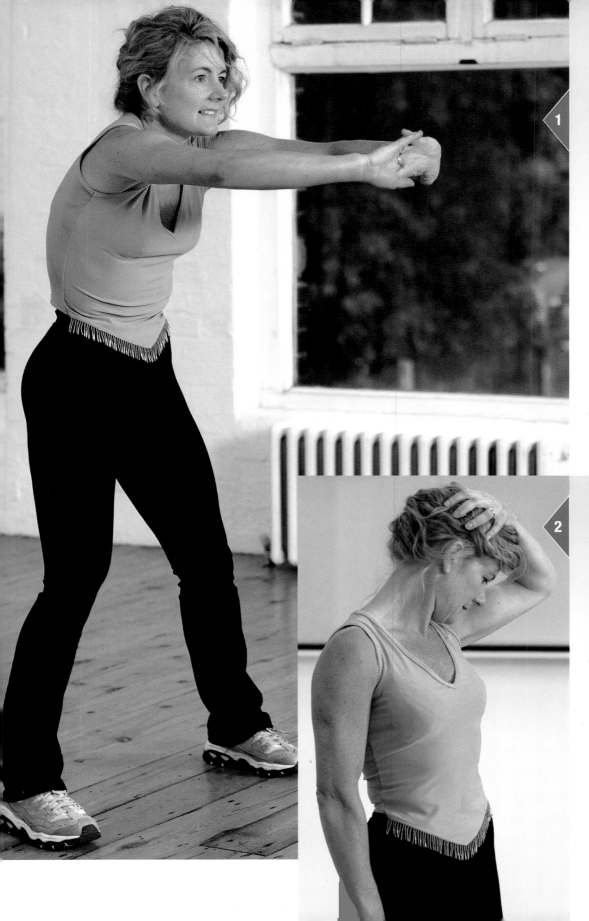

1

Upper-back Stretch

Stand with your feet shoulder-distance apart and knees soft. Pull your abs towards your backbone and reach your arms out in front of you, rounding out your spine.

2

Neck and Spine Stretch

Stand with your knees soft. With your left arm at your side and shoulders relaxed, slowly bend your chin to your chest and turn towards your right shoulder. Place your right hand on your head and gently stretch away from your left shoulder. Repeat on the other side.

Side Stretch

Stand with your feet shoulder-distance apart and knees soft. With your hands clasped overhead, slightly twist your torso to the right. Now stretch further by pressing your hands away from your body whilst focusing on keeping the rib cage stationary. Repeat on the other side.

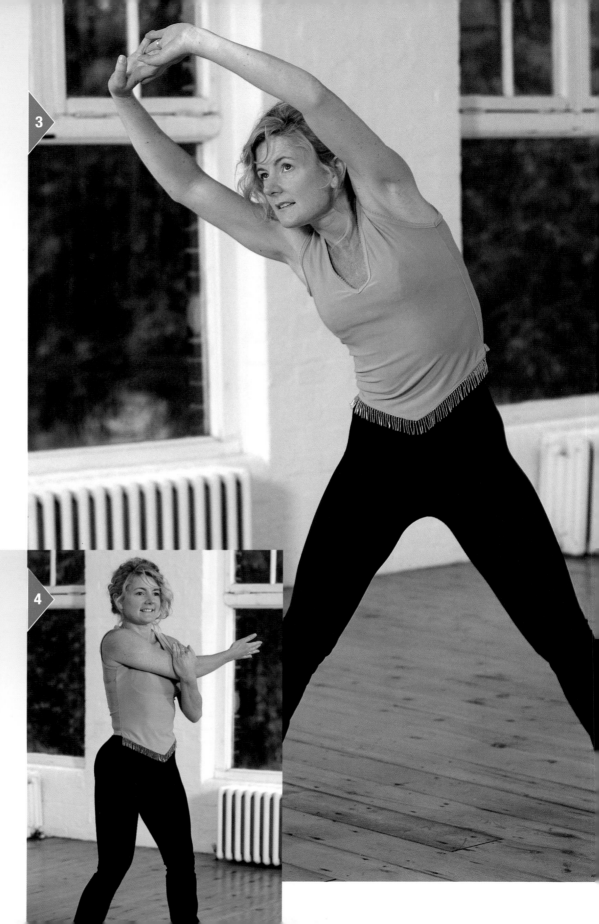

Rear-shoulder Stretch

Stand with your feet together and knees soft. Gently pull your right arm across your torso by applying pressure above your elbow with your left hand. Do not allow your torso to twist as you pull your arm across.

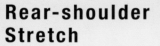

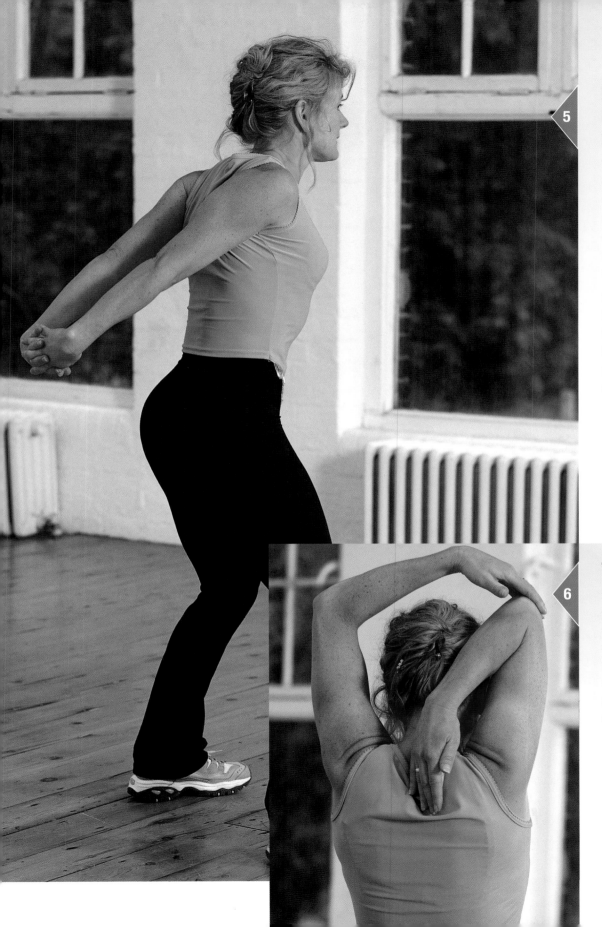

5

Front-shoulder, Chest and Biceps Stretch

This stretch is important for improving posture. By regularly working the back muscles, stretching and opening out the chest muscles, the bust will appear to have lifted due to the shoulders being pulled back.

Stand with your feet together, knees soft and pelvis tilted forward. Clasp your hands behind your back. Keeping your position stable lift your arms up and away from your body.

6

Triceps Stretch

Standing with your feet together and knees soft. Take one arm overhead, bending your elbow so your hand touches between your shoulder blades. Take your other hand and gently push your elbow with it. Repeat on the other side.

All-over Back Release

Stand with your legs apart and knees bent. Lean forwards and place your hands on your thighs (not your knees). Keeping the lower body stationary, with a straight back drop your right shoulder towards your left knee. Repeat on the other side.

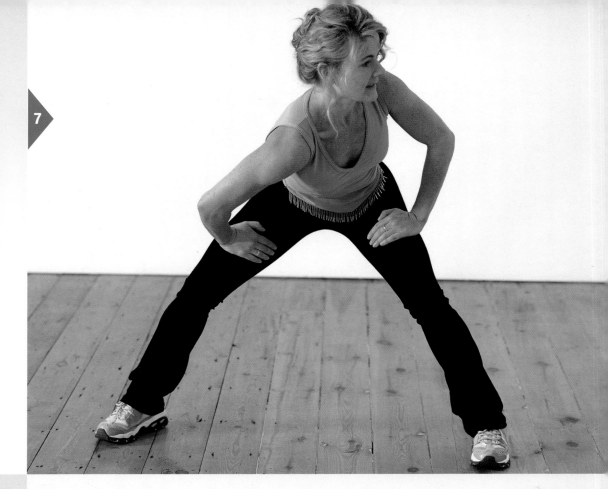

Hip Flexor Stretch

Many of us have tight hip flexors which is often linked to back pain. Rugby players are renowned for having tight hip flexor muscles due to the amount of kicking they do. However, these muscles also tighten up through sitting at a desk all day. The tightness causes the back muscles to take the strain. So for those of you sitting at a desk all day – do this stretch regularly.

Come into a deep lunge position making sure you have a right angle with your front knee. Place one hand on the floor and the other on your thigh. Keep your back straight. Repeat on the other side.

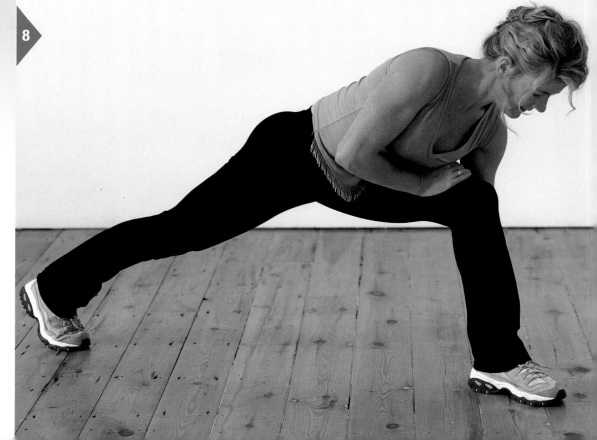

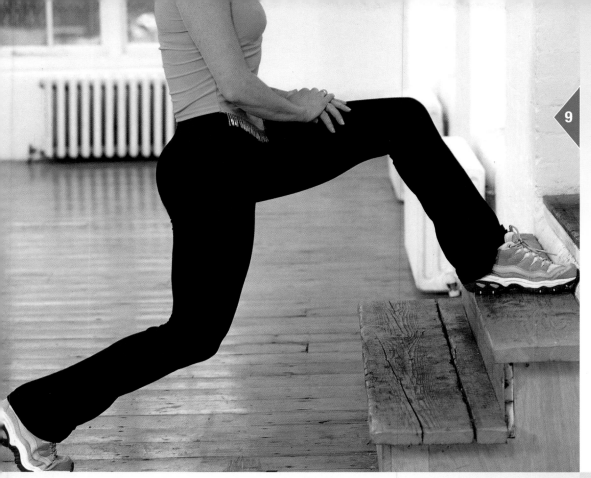

Intensive Hip Flexor Stretch

9

This stretch works well and you can immediately feel its intensity. Many people fail to identify with this muscle but once mastered you really can understand its origin. You'll know when you're stretching this muscle.

Standing at the bottom of a staircase, place your left foot on the 2nd or 3rd step. Take a step back with your right foot, lift your heel off the floor, tilt your pelvis and lower your right knee towards the floor. Hold and repeat on the other side.

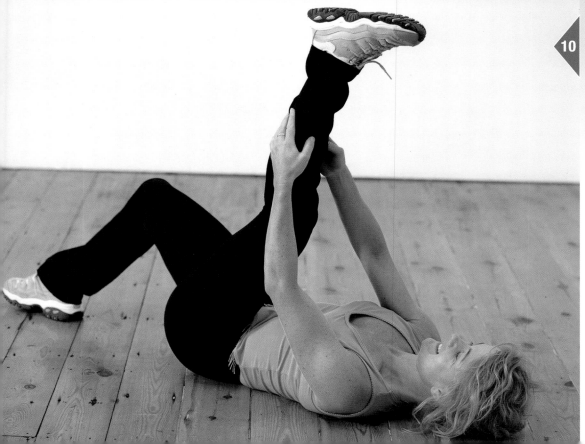

Hamstring Stretch

10

Lie on your back, knees bent and feet on the floor. Extend one foot up towards the ceiling and hold behind your calf. Do not lift your hip off the floor, let it sink down and keep the knee slightly bent. Repeat on the other side.

Calf Stretch

This is an important stretch particularly if you frequently wear high heels.

Stand on the edge of a step and hold onto a support. Keeping your left foot on the step, bring the ball of your right foot to the edge of the step. Press the heel down until you feel the stretch. Repeat on the other side.

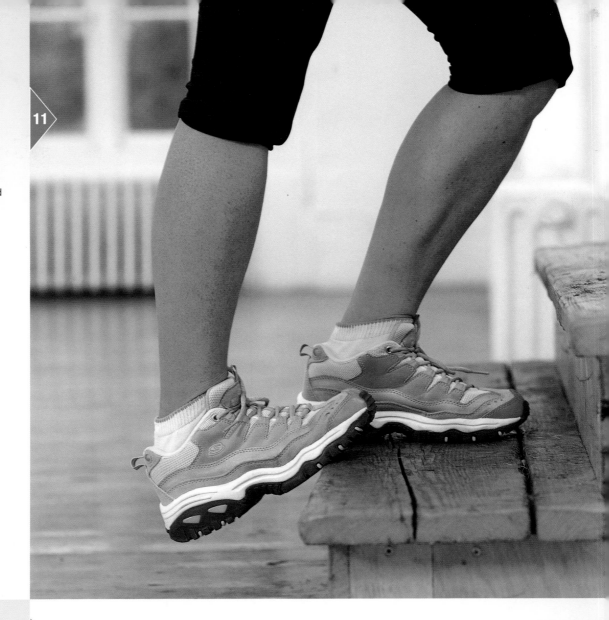

Quad Stretch

Lie on your stomach and place your head on one hand. With the other hand pull your foot up to your buttock making sure your hips remain pressed down. Repeat on the other side.

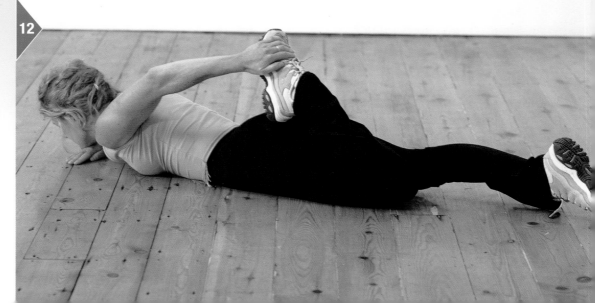

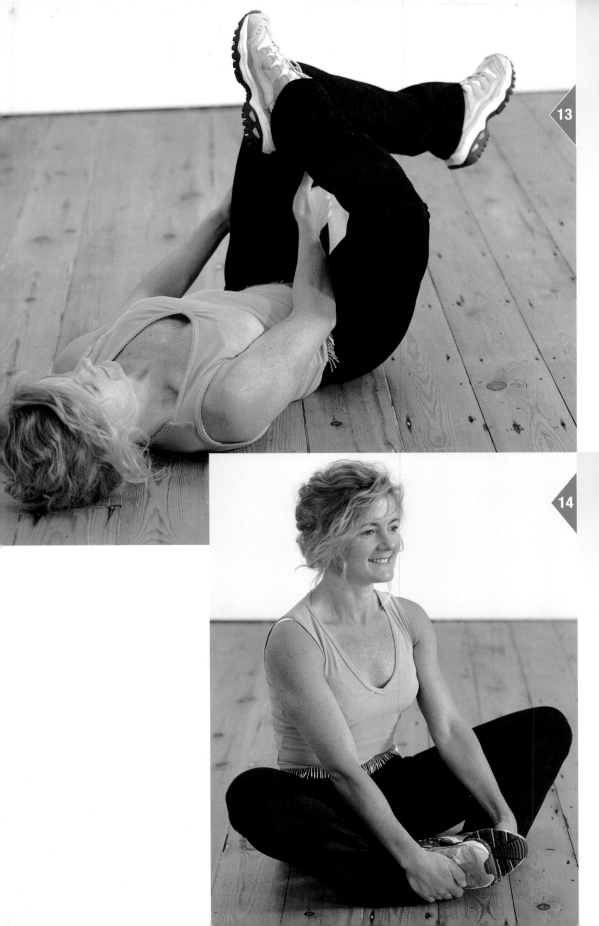

13

Buttock Stretch

Lie on your back with your knees bent. Place your right foot on your left knee. Lift your left foot off the floor and draw your knee towards you. Push your right knee outward. Repeat on the other side.

14

Inner-thigh Stretch

Sitting on the floor, put the soles of your shoes together and draw your feet up to the centre of your body. Keeping your back straight and holding your feet, gently push your knees down towards the floor and hold.

Outer-thigh and Back Stretch

Sitting, extend your left leg out
in front of you and place your
right foot over your extended
leg. Keeping your back straight,
twist your torso to the right and
place your left arm on your
right leg. Look over your
right shoulder. Repeat on
the other side.

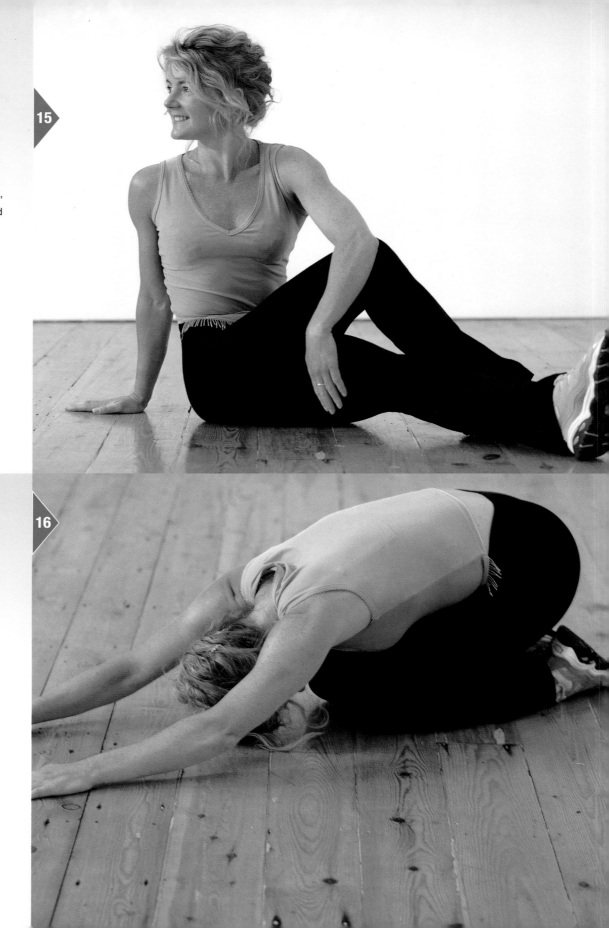

Stretching on all fours

Sit back on your heels and
walk your fingers as far
forward as you can without
lifting your buttocks.

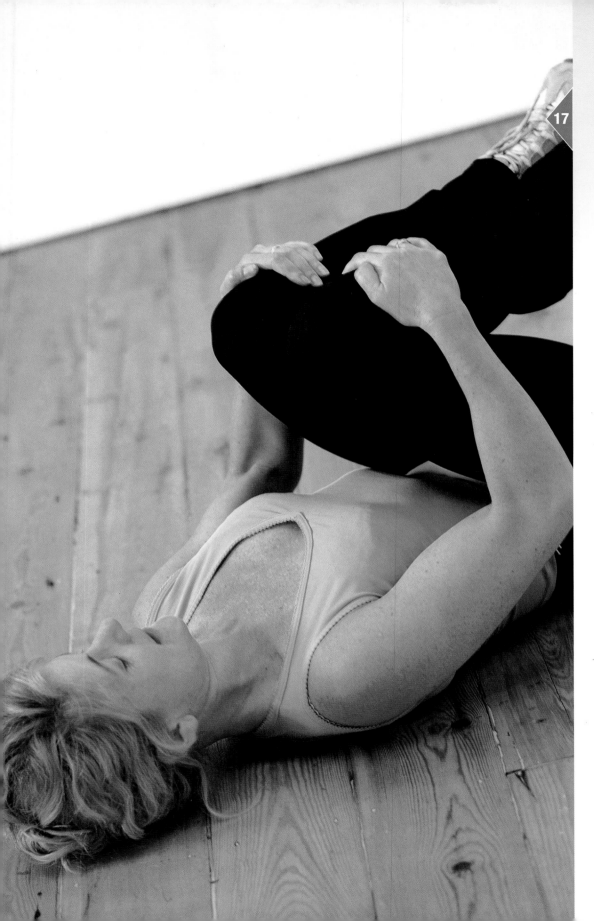

17

Lower-back Stretch

Lie on your back, pull your knees into your chest and gently rock from side to side. Now holding your knees snugly, circle 4 times to the right and 4 times to the left.

WORKOUTS
THAT WORK

- *Commit time to exercise*
- *Challenge yourself outdoors*
- *Indoor workout wonders*

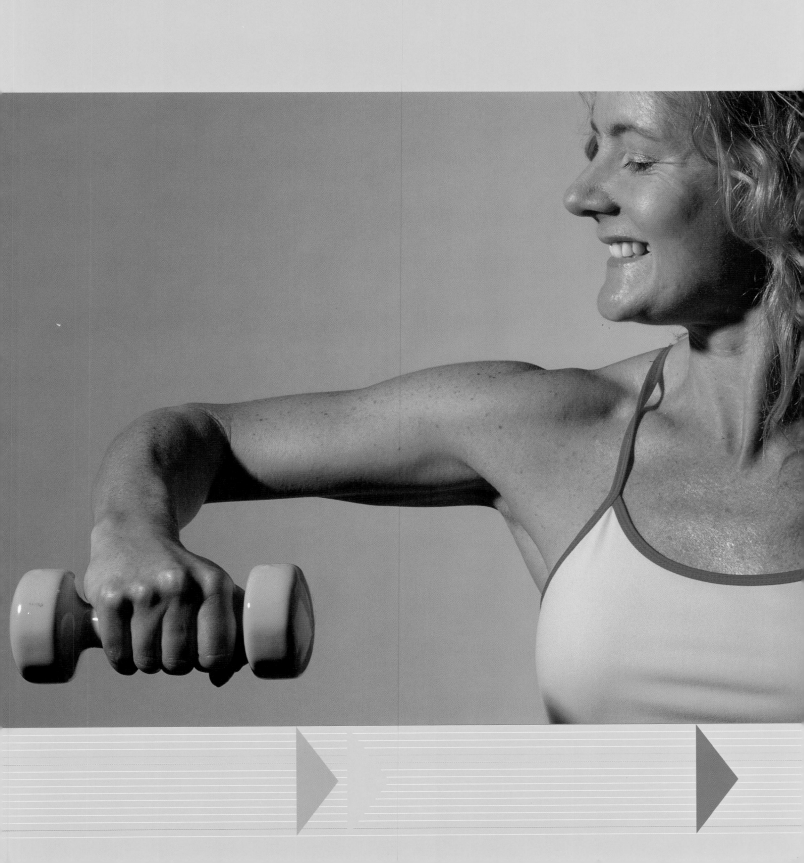

WORKOUTS

Time to revamp your exercise programme and burn more calories by creating more variety and intensity into your existing routines. It's called progression. Part of the reason many of us give up on exercise is through boredom, which is not surprising especially when your weight hits those dreadful plateaus. By supplementing your routines with these specially designed workouts, you will almost double the amount of calories you are burning. Part of the effectiveness is that you are constantly giving the mind and body new stimuli and obstacles to overcome.

Douglas Brooks, one of the world's most renowned fitness consultants, says: 'Committing time to exercise is critical,' and he advocates changing your workouts regularly. 'By tracking your progress, and keeping your workouts time-efficient and results-orientated you will be able to accomplish your health and fitness goals.'

Alternatively, if you are on the brink of giving up exercise due to lack of time, then do not despair. I have all the answers! Why is it that we assume 'real' fitness has to be characterised by lengthy vigorous workouts that last no less than 60 minutes. Perhaps we have this image of Demi Moore or Madonna, both of whom are known to overdo it in the exercise department. My work with the Princess of Wales showed that quality was far superior to quantity. The beautifully sculpted body she attained was achieved with just three workouts per week. This was occasionally supplemented with tennis and swimming.

So, if lack of time is your excuse for not exercising, that's all it is, an excuse. Fitting a couple of 10-minute walks into your day or using the stairs instead of the lift would go a long way to improving your overall fitness level.

The American College of Sports Medicine recommends 20–60 continuous or accumulated minutes of aerobic exercise every day. Add two to three sessions of strength and flexibility training each week and you have a complete fitness programme.

The message, clearly, is to get started on a regular fitness programme and stick with it. Occasionally, when only one workout a week has been permissible, be sure to fit three or four sessions in the following week. In fact, studies have shown that if you reduced frequency and endurance but sustained intensity whilst training, there would be no decrease in oxygen consumption, for up to 15 weeks. In layman's terms, it's okay to miss one or two sessions from time to time. When you do get the chance to exercise make sure it is intensive enough to make up for other losses. Whether you are going on a business trip, having guests to stay, or going on holiday always plan exercise into your schedule just as you would pack your toothbrush.

Here are a variety of ideas and workouts to keep your fitness goals focused during disruptive periods or to give your existing workouts a boost. With consistent exercise you can change the shape of your body in 8–12 weeks.

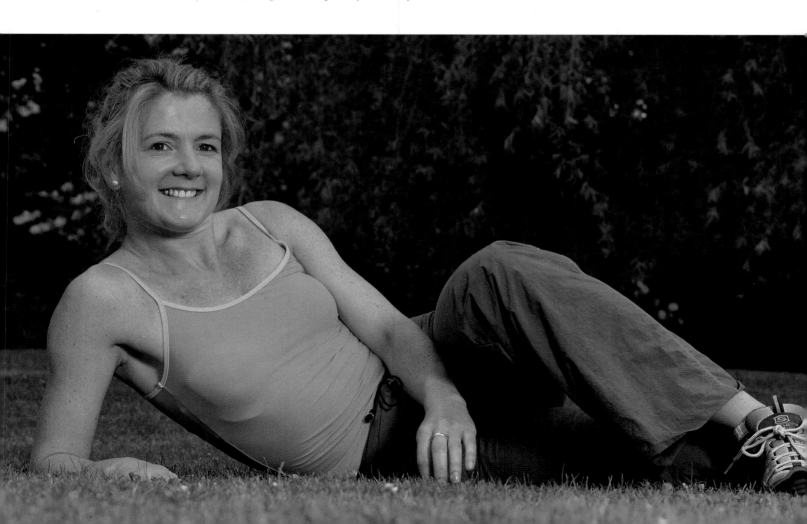

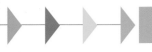

Great outdoor workouts

Need to shed that winder padding? Want to break bad eating habits? Need to elimate stress? Get yourself out of the house and do these great workouts. You'll be amazed with the results.

These two workouts have been devised as challenging, time-efficient and fun. The aim is to bump up your fat-burning exercise routine. If your goal is to lose extra body fat, do either of these routines at least four times a week for best results. Alternatively, you could alternate them. Once completed you'll feel ready to conquer any mountain! Choose an inspiring safe area near your home to work out.

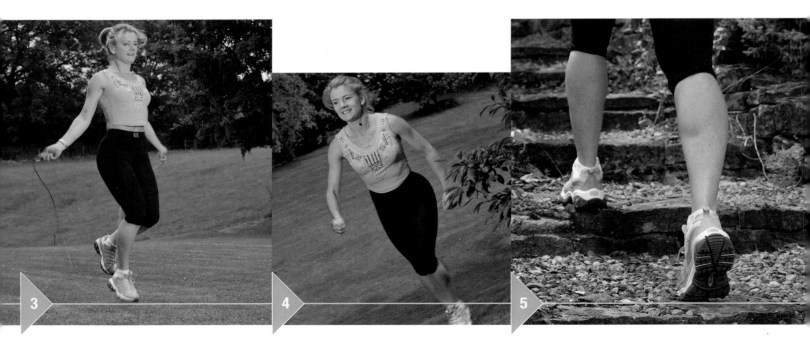

3

Skip

For 5 minutes. Keep the pace going. Alternate single and double foot jumps.

4

Power walk

For another 10 minutes with your heart rate in the fat-burning zone.

5

Climb stairs

For 5 minutes. Walk briskly up and down a set of stairs.

Workout 1

This routine, in particular, is great for burning fat and getting rid of any post Christmas weight. Aim to do this four times a week for maximum results.

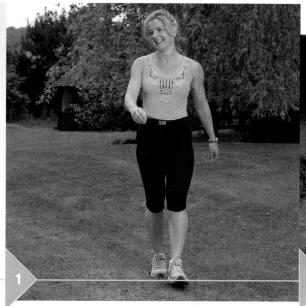

1

Warm up

Start out with 7–10 minutes walking, including a few warm-up stretches.

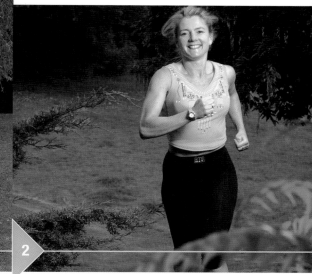

2

Power walk

For 10 minutes. Keep your heart rate at the top end of your fat-burning zone.

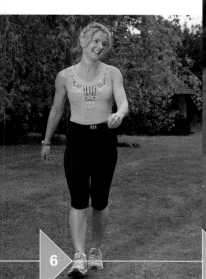

6

Cool down

For 5 minutes by walking slowly.

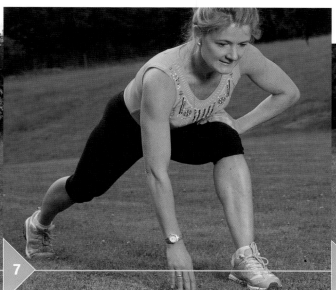

7

Stretch

Do some lower-body stretches.

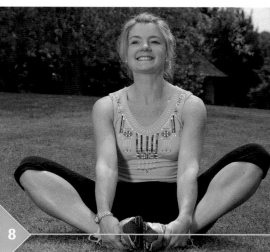

8

Stretch

Workout 2

This routine is the more challenging of the two and the cross training will shape up your body quickly. When you are power walking (step 2) try to make sure your heart rate is being challenged by keeping it in the fat-burning zone and higher. Once you have reached the halfway point stop and do exercise steps 3–7 before power walking the other way.

Keep going without a break if you can.

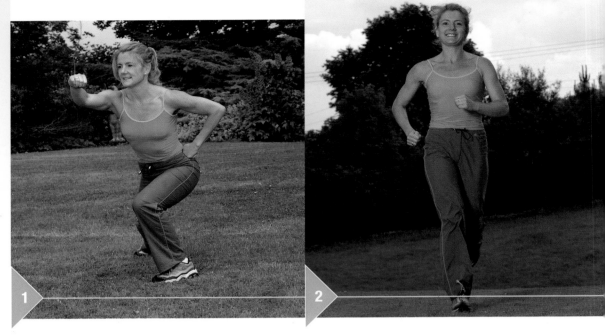

Warm up

Start out with 7–10 minutes walking, including a few warm-up stretches.

Power walk or jog

For 15 or 20 minutes in one direction.

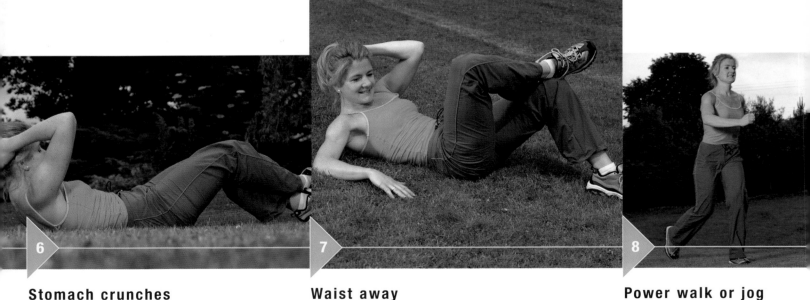

Stomach crunches

20 reps (see p.94).

Waist away

16 reps each side (see p.99). Note that in this exercise the foot is placed on the knee.

Power walk or jog

For 15–20 minutes the other way.

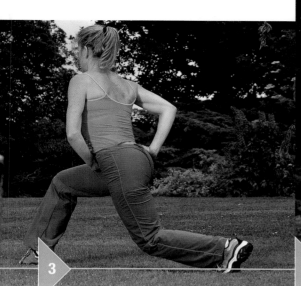

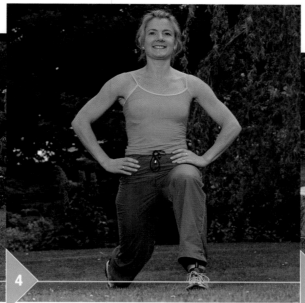

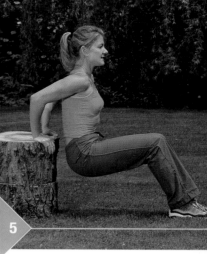

Crossover reverse behind

Do 10 reps with the right leg then go on to step 4 (see p.73).

Reverse lunge

Do 10 reps with the right leg then repeat steps 3 and 4 with the left leg (see p.72).

Triceps dips

10 reps, 2 sets (see p.51).

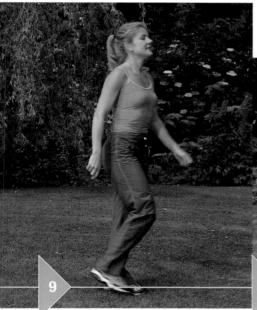

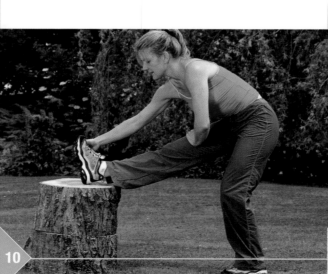

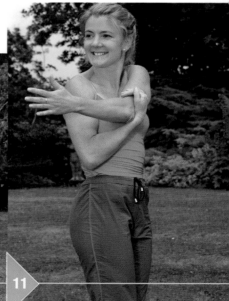

Cool down

Walk for 3 minutes.

Stretches

For the lower body.

Stretches

For the upper body (see p.102-105).

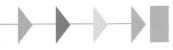

Fifteen-minute workout wonders

You've been meaning to do your workout all day but got side tracked. The kids still have to be fed and you're due to meet up with friends. Rushed off your feet, you feel guilty and angry for not having done some exercise. Here are two very effective routines for you to choose from. Because each routine lasts only 15 minutes, work out with weights of 2–3kg. This extra load will force the muscles to work harder. Because you are only using these routines as 'fill-ins' there is no chance of bulking up. Keep moving from one exercise to the next to keep the heart rate up as much as possible. As always, it is extremely important to maintain perfect quality through each move for maximum benefit. Although these routines only take 15 minutes they will leave you feeling like you've had an hour's workout and psychologically a whole lot better for having done something too.

Once you have warmed up do exercises two through to seven, then repeat them before stretching.

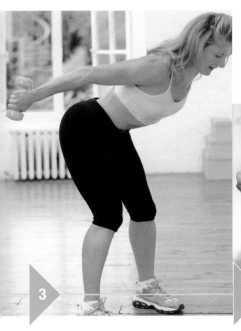

3

Triceps extensions

15 reps (see p.54).

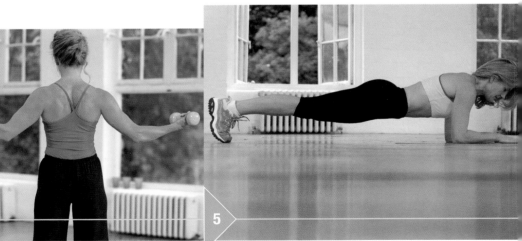

4

Super-shapely back

15 reps (see p.65).

5

Bridge

Repeat 5 times (see p.100).

Workout 3

This workout focuses on women's problem areas whilst still being time-efficient.

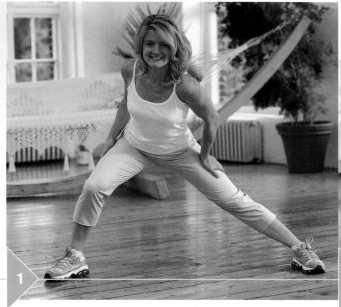

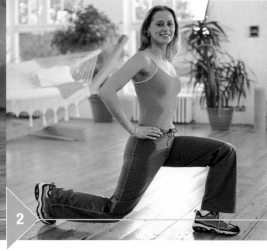

Warm up

For 5 minutes to your favourite music. Marching or low impact moves are ideal.

Lunge for lean and lovely legs

8 alternate lunges in one direction, and 8 in the opposite direction (see p.74).

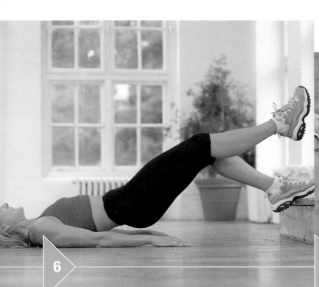

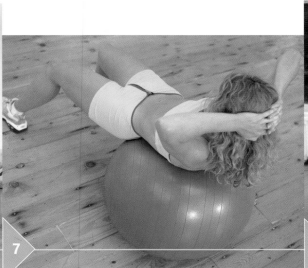

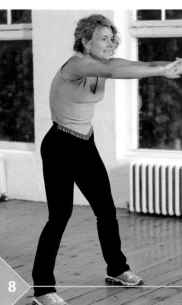

Hamstring and butt buster

12 times each side (see p.88).

Crunch with the ball

Repeat 20 reps (see p.96).

Stretch

(see p.103)

Workout 4

This workout is a little more challenging and will certainly get your heart rate up. It is quick, fun and very effective.

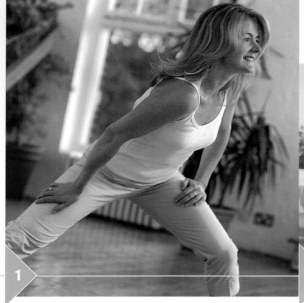

Warm up

For 5 minutes to your favourite music. Marching or low-impact dance moves.

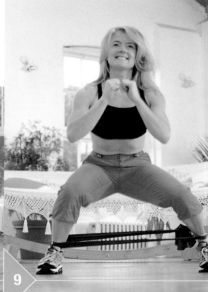

Warm-up stretches

(see p.48–49)

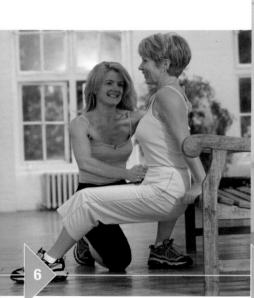

Tricep dips

Repeat 12 reps (see p.51).

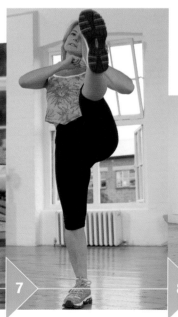

Kick butt

10 reps on each side.
(see p.77)

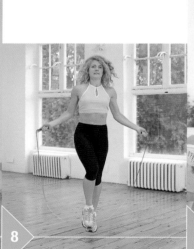

Skip

For 2 minutes.

Alternate leg squats with dynaband

12 alternate reps, 2 sets (see p.79)

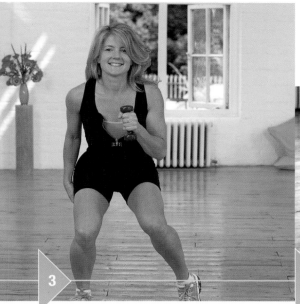

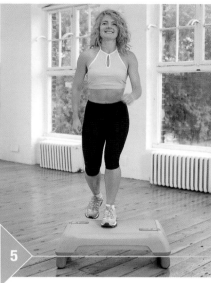

3

Squat and abduct

Repeat 10 times on each side (see p.75). Add strong tricep extensions.

4

Reverse lunge

12 reps with each leg. (see p.72). With each lunge behind add a bicep curl.

5

Step up

For 2 minutes.

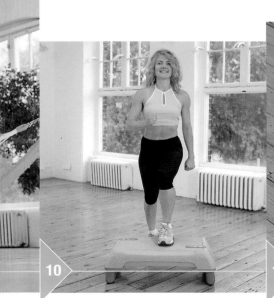

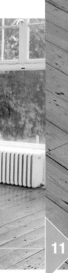

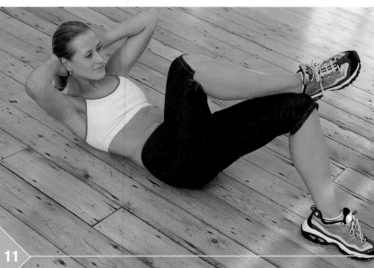

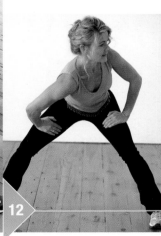

10

Step up

For 2 minutes.

11

Lift and circle

Repeat 12 reps each way (see p.98).

12

Stretch

(see p.106)

Diet and
METABOLISM

- *Eat regularly and do not yo-yo diet or binge*

- *Choose foods that increase your metabolic rate*

- *Avoid saturated fats and sugars*

- *Exercise aerobically and strength train regularly*

- *Do not over-exercise and under-eat*

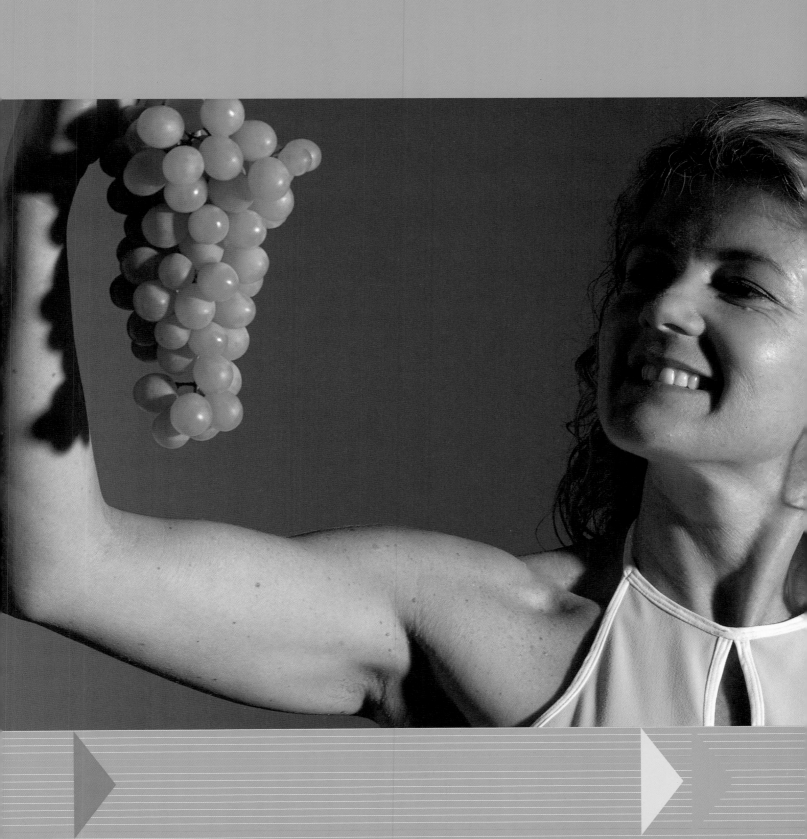

YOUR METABOLISM

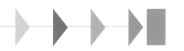

I have been in the very fortunate position of having gained more than 20 pounds which on my small frame was quite excessive. Yes, fortunate, because it really gave me an insight into the feelings of being overweight and the emotions involved with it. Growing up with a mother who had a perfect figure after giving birth to six children seemed like a hard act to follow, especially when I reached my late teens and was repeatedly told that I had more than likely inherited my father's side of the family genes which are bottom heavy.

> *Next to genes, lifestyle habits are the biggest shapers of the human body.*

With no experience in nutrition or exercise at all I decided to prove them all wrong. Little did I realise, at the time, that this would cost me nearly ten years of dieting and being unhappy with my body shape. I tried every new diet in the book and was exercising like mad. My situation was desperate. I set about finding the solution and have not looked back since. I know there are millions of you out there in similar positions, and my aim is to help save you from years of unpleasant memories about your body shape by providing you with the right information to transform yourself.

Genes are what we inherit from our ancestors. Studies show that your weight is 70% genetic. That leaves an important 30% in your hands and getting the balance between exercise and diet is crucial. Richard Cotton, chief exercise physiologist at the American Council on Exercise (ACE), agrees, saying that although diet, cardiovascular conditioning and strength training significantly influence body size and shape, genetics is the number one factor. Having taken control of my 30% has prevented me from claiming my father's genes, and now everyone tells me that I have my mother's genes. Hmmm!

Rev up your metabolism

Research shows that over time, you can permanently raise your metabolism by up to 8% – burning an extra 700 calories or so per week. Metabolism is the amount of energy expended by the body on a daily basis just to maintain homeostasis, or the basic amount of energy required to survive without any extra activity. This accounts for 60% of our daily calorie expenditure. The faster your metabolic rate, the more efficient your fat-burning pathways will be. Your metabolism is the key factor to long-term weight loss.

Factors Affecting Metabolism

• Toned muscles will significantly increase your RMR.

• A woman's hormonal system resists changes in body composition as a protective mechanism that helps conserve energy during pregnancy. Women, therefore, lose fat at a slower rate than men and find it difficult to maintain very low body-fat levels. Men have a higher metabolic rate than women and this is largely due to the fact that they have more muscle mass.

• The more active you are, the faster your RMR will be. If you study people who are generally lean and not dieters, you will notice that they are active people.

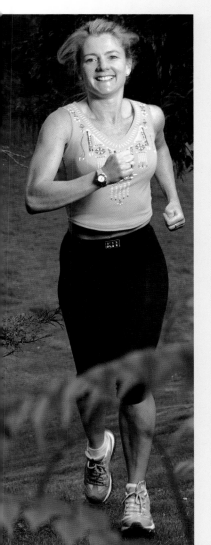

• Smoking has an increasing effect on metabolic rate. Weight gain can occur after giving up but this is usually due to smokers eating more to fill the void.

• Your metabolism favours a regular eating plan. Yo-yo dieting causes the metabolism to slow right down to enable it to cope with those famine weeks.

• Research shows that adults experience a gradual decrease in resting metabolism of about 3.2–5.0% per decade. Exercise and proper eating habits can and will slow this reduction down dramatically.

• From repeated bouts of dieting many women are in danger of taking this situation to the extremes. Through fear of regaining weight, they become obsessive, many cutting calories to less than 1000 per day and spending hours exercising. Initially this causes weight loss but sustaining this pattern for some time causes the body to lower its metabolic set point in an effort to conserve energy. The end result is weight gain.

• Studies show that the RMR stays elevated for up to 18 hours after aerobic activity.

DIET– Don't It Ends in Tears

By now you should be afraid of even mentioning the D word! Since my formula does not advocate dieting, I am not going to give you a diet to follow. The goal is not to lose a certain number of pounds in a certain number of weeks or months but to reach a reduced body-fat percentage that is both realistic and achievable within your time constraints. Therefore, I aim to educate you about food and where you have gone wrong in the past, giving you a set of guidelines to help you on your way to a leaner, fitter and healthier body. Once you have given your body a fair chance to adapt to these changes they will become permanent.

GMTV host Lorraine Kelly, who had been on every kind of diet until she met me, sums it up perfectly: 'Working with Jenni was the first time I had combined proper eating with exercise and stuck to the programme.' She has now maintained her svelte new look for almost two years. 'Although I do go off track from time to time,' says Lorraine 'it is wonderful not to go to bed at night dreaming about my breakfast the next morning.'

Congratulations if you have made the decision to abandon dieting forever. Great! You can start eating food without ever having to feel guilty again. From now on you are going to eat three healthy meals a day with snacks in between. We know the metabolism favours this formula. Make the decision to eat these healthy meals from Monday to Friday and on the weekend endeavour to continue eating healthily and if you do happen to go off track, don't allow it to become a downward spiral and don't let it turn into a binge. By becoming an intuitive eater you will stop eating when you feel satisfied which could mean not quite finishing your desert. You will only eat when you are hungry and you will find yourself reaching more towards healthy, energy-giving food, rather than the junk food that previously dominated your diet. Allow your body to start healing itself first and then you'll be motivated to carry on and weight loss will follow.

> *You can start eating food without ever having to feel guilty again.*

Sticking to this plan is surprisingly easy once you realise it does work. The choice is yours. Either stop yo-yo dieting now and give your body a chance to re-adjust, or spend the rest of your life trying out the latest diet. I know which one I would choose.

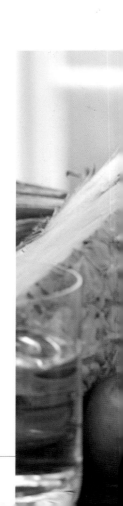

The Jenergy diet

We are going to turn your body into a fat-burning furnace that keeps ticking over at a steady pace. Healthy eating involves a variety of food, a wholesome diet and eating with moderation. Variety is key to making sure your body has an adequate supply of all the nutrients it needs. When the body lacks certain nutrients, cravings often set in and send us running for the very thing we shouldn't have. Eating too much of the same type of food everyday has been known to cause an allergic reaction to that food. Ensure that you eat fresh fruit and vegetables at least once, preferably twice a day. Choose wholewheat over white bread and buy ingredients to make your own sauces rather than buying packaged sauces.

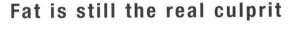

Eating with moderation means trying to ensure that at least 80% of your diet is healthy. If you stick to this principle consistently, then even a sausage sandwich or an ice-cream can fit into a well-balanced diet. You'll be amazed how the body deals with junk food provided you learn to get right back on track.

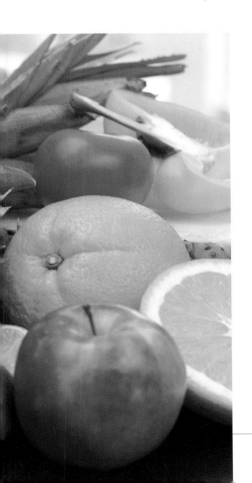

Fat is still the real culprit

The Pritikan diet was one of the first to advocate low-fat eating, not only to lose weight but to help prevent cancer and heart disease. This was how I first became interested in nutrition and lost my weight. Then the whole dieting industry jumped onto the 'low-fat' bandwagon. Almost every packaged food was branded low-fat. It was taken to extremes. Many women were cutting fat totally from their diets. Or, if they weren't totally cutting the fat they were buying packets of non-fat biscuits and devouring the whole packet at one sitting. Both of these behavioural patterns caused illness, hormonal disturbances, dry skin, hair and nails and many other unpleasant symptoms.

After years of low-fat living the pendulum swung the other way and suddenly everyone was being told that fat was not in fact the culprit and to balance the ratio of fat, carbohydrate and protein. Being told fat was on the menu again was not a smart idea because slowly but surely it has crept back into our diets in a big way.

You've guessed. We're eating too much bad fat and not enough good fat. Simply correct this imbalance and don't be lured into high-protein, low-carbohydrate diets. Don't mix this or that type of diet that will only disappoint you.

We burn about 60 calories of fat per hour at night which equals 480 calories of fat if we sleep an eight-hour night. Remember, we have an unlimited supply of fat which is the prime fuel used as energy throughout the day. Therefore a shortage of fat is hardly likely.

Fat in your diet

Too much fat in the diet plays an enormous role in the development and progression of many diseases such as obesity, high blood pressure, high cholesterol, liver, kidney and heart disease, bowel and breast cancer, arthritis, gout and strokes. One of the prime reasons we're consuming too much fat is because there are so many hidden fats in the food we eat nowadays. Even products which claim to be low fat have cleverly found ways to trick the consumer. You'll learn to discover hidden fats and how to work out the fat grams in all products.

We have an unlimited supply of fat which is the prime fuel used as energy throughout the day.

Fat is also tasty and one of the reasons why going on a fad diet is so counter productive. After a week of just cabbages or bananas, our bodies are crying out for some comforting tasty food. Food laden with sauces normally does the trick and before you know it you're consuming a whopping 100g of fat or more a day . . . again! In reality you really have not given your body the chance to stick to a healthy amount of fat on a regular basis. Now is the time to do that.

How much fat is healthy?

In order to maintain health and prevent diseases it is generally accepted in medical fields that no more than 30% of your calories should derive from fat. Most of us consume far more than that – up to 50%. To lose fat we need to cut it out of our diets as best we can. I suggest for healthy weight loss you aim to eat between 20–25% fat per day. Once you reach your goal weight try to stick to no more than 25% fat per day.

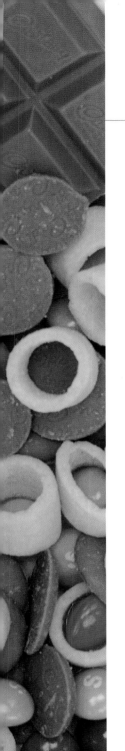

How to calculate the fat in your diet

Once you know this simple formula there should be no excuse for you not to adhere to a low-fat eating plan. If you're an active woman who eats about 2,000 calories per day, 500 calories of these could come from fat, or 25%:

2,000 calories x 25% fat = 500 calories from fat

There are 9 calories in 1g fat, to work out how many fat grams this is:

500 (calories) divided by 9(g) = 55g

Knowing that you can eat up to 55g of fat per day is very helpful when you learn how much fat is in different foods. As a guide eat 35–45g of fat a day for weight loss and 45–55g for weight control. By rationing your intake of butter, margarine, mayonnaise, salad dressings, crisps, ice cream, cookies and other obviously high-fat foods, you will be consuming about a 25% fat diet.

Calorie needs per day	Grams of fat for 25% fat intake
1,200	35g
1,500	40g
1,800	50g
2,000	55g
2,200	60g

Read the food labels and find the fat

We see them plastered on almost every product in the supermarkets in an attempt to lure us into buying them: diet, lite, lo-cal, slimmer's, low-fat, no-fat. When buying products always read the label on the back. First of all read the list of ingredients. These should be listed in descending order from the largest ingredient to the smallest. To work out the percentage of fat read the 'Typical Nutrition Information'. Let's say there are 14.7g of fat in a 40g bag of crisps. If we multiply this by nine (because there are nine calories in every gram of fat) we get 132 calories of fat. The total calories in a bag of crisps in 213. Therefore, the percentage of fat calories is a whopping 60% fat. By being aware of your daily allowance you will not exceed that limit.

Additionally, be wary of the so-called 'healthy' branding on many products. The manufacturers may call a product healthy even if it only has one healthy ingredient in it, despite the fact that it's loaded with fat and sugar.

Fat grams in some common foods

Food Source	Quantity	Fat grams
Dairy		
Milk – full fat	250ml (1cup)	10g
Milk – skim	250ml (1cup)	0g
Cheddar cheese	25g (1oz)	10g
Mozzarella	25g (1oz)	7g
Cottage cheese	25g (1oz)	2g
Yogurt – full-fat	250ml (1cup)	8g
Yogurt – low-fat	250ml (1cup)	4g
Butter	20g (1tbsp)	11g
Margarine	20g (1tbsp)	15g
Ice cream (16%+ fat)	55g (½cup)	15g
Ice cream (10% fat)	55g (½cup)	5g
Lean meats/fish (trimmed & cooked)		
Chicken	115g (4oz)	5g
Lamb	115g (4oz)	11g
Beef	115g (4oz)	14g
Pork	115g (4oz)	15g
Tuna		
(canned in water)	115g (4oz)	2g
Salmon	115g (4oz)	15g
Halibut	115g (4oz)	9g
Bacon – grilled	2strips	7g

Food Source	Quantity	Fat grams
Nuts and seeds		
Almonds	12	10g
Brazil nuts	50g (2oz)	35g
Cashew nuts	50g (2oz)	26g
Peanuts – roasted sesame, pumpkin	75g (3oz)	35g
Sunflower seeds	30g (1oz)	14g
Other foods		
Olive oil	50ml (¼cup)	54g
Vegetable oil	20ml (1tbsp)	15g
Mayonnaise	20ml (1tbsp)	10g
Eggs – boiled or poached	1	6g
Fried eggs	1	8g
Avocado	½ medium	18g
Junk/fast foods		
French fries	1cup	10g
Sausage – fried	1medium	10g
Croissant	1medium	14g
Hamburger	¼ pounder	23g
Pizza (cheese and tomato)	1 average slice	10g

What fats should I be eating?

Specific fats are essential to your health, and play a crucial role in protecting you from a range of disorders. These are essential fatty acids (EFAs). For example, oily fish. This is a subject I feel strongly about, and precisely where the Jenergy low-fat principles differ from other low-fat hip and thigh diets, which treat all fats as equal, including oils, oily fish, seeds, egg yolks and avocados. Our bodies need EFAs for balanced hormonal function, for supple skin and arteries, for nerve cell insulation, for prevention of joint pain and inflammation, and to keep warm. Interestingly, EFAs can also increase metabolic rate thereby stimulating increased weight loss.

By knowing that you should include a certain amount of fat in your diet it's easy to pick and choose which fats you want to include in your daily allowance. For example, why waste your allowance of fat grams on a 40g packet of crisps laden with 14.7g of fat. Instead you could have eaten one third of an avocado in a salad sandwich worth about 12g of fat. Although avocados are high in fat it is a healthy fat, which provided fits into your daily allowance, will actually do more good than harm. To make sure you are getting an adequate intake of EFAs try to follow these recommendations:

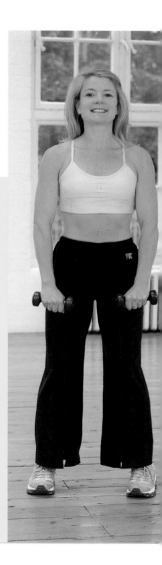

Essential fatty acids

- Eat oily fish such as mackerel, sardines and salmon.

- Use extra virgin olive oil for cooking.

- Other suggested oils such as sesame, sunflower or safflower are great for salads. Make sure they are unrefined and cold pressed.

- Use butter in moderation and instead of margarine.

- Eat nuts (almonds, walnuts, hazelnuts and pecans) and seeds (sesame, sunflower and pumpkin) in moderation.

- Eat avocados in moderation.

- To ensure your body receives an adequate amount of EFAs take a stable fish oil supplement and/or evening primrose, borage or blackcurrant seed oil.

- Make sure these essential fats are included in your daily fat gram allowance.

Protein

Protein sources should account for 15–20% of your diet. For most women this equates to about 60–75g per day, taking in the higher range if you are more active. By learning to read food labels you can easily assess whether you are meeting your protein needs or not. For example, there are 25g of protein in a 200g tin of water-packed tuna and 5.9g of protein in a 125g pot of yogurt. Protein is essential for building and repairing muscles, red blood cells, hair, and other tissues. Our body can provide some of the amino acids which make up protein but we have to get other amino acids from our diet. To make sure you get all essential amino acids, eat high-protein foods such as meat, poultry and fish. Choose lean meats and skinless chicken, turkey and fish. Eggs are a good source of protein but also high in fat so limit them to 2–3 per week.

Carbohydrates

Unfortunately, misconceptions about carbohydrates and weight prevent many people from making good carbohydrate selections. There are two types of carbohydrates: simple and complex. Cut back on complex carbohydrates only minimally, since they help maintain the blood-sugar level and provide a steady supply of energy.

Complex	Simple
Grains (wheat, oats, rye, rice, maize, barley)	Fruit
	Sugar (white and brown)
Pulses (lentils, beans, chickpeas)	Honey
	Biscuits
Vegetables	Cakes

Carbohydrates are the best choice for fuelling your muscles and when present in the diet, the body burns fat more efficiently. Carbohydrates are not fattening! Fats are fattening, and many protein foods also contain a lot of fat. Carbohydrates become fattening when you add hefty doses of fat, such as butter on bread and sour cream on potatoes. Complex carbohydrates should acccount for 50–60% of your daily diet, and when choosing these, go for the unrefined carbohydrates. For example, choose wholewheat bread, brown rice and wholemeal flour instead of the white refined versions, which have been stripped of essential nutrients. Aim to keep simple carbohydrates to a minimum.

The calories you subtract from your diet should come first from dietary fats, then from simple carbohydrates, and finally from complex carbohydrates. These three calorie sources are the fat-causing culprits. By cutting down drastically on carbohydrates you are ultimately going on a high-protein diet. High-protein diets cause muscle and water to be lost, not fat.

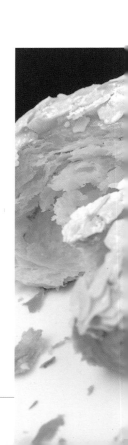

Sugar

Eating sugar occasionally will not adversely affect the body in any way. It certainly will not cause weight gain. With a fit, metabolically charged body, sugar in small doses or even the odd binge, will go unnoticed. We know that sugar stimulates the release of insulin, which encourages fat storage and most sugary products such as biscuits and chocolates are loaded with fat. Therefore eating too much sugar can cause weight gain. To control insulin you must control the intake of sugar, both the refined variety and sugars found in many carbohydrates.

There is a method of measuring the impact of food on our blood-sugar levels, known as the Glycemic Index. This is a guide and circumstances vary from person to person depending on their state of health 'right now'. By following the Jenergy principles blood-sugar levels should stabilise, as well as the body's ability to tolerate carbohydrates.

As a guide, it is recommended that we eat foods that have a Glycemic Index of 64 or below. Foods over 70 should be kept to a minimum or combined with foods of a lower Glycemic Index number.

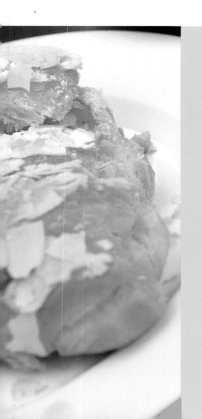

The Glycemic Index

Fruit		Pulses		Grains and cereals	
Banana	62	Baked beans	48	Bagel	72
Apple	39	Kidney beans	29	White bread	70
Orange	40	Butter beans	36	Wholewheat bread	46
Melon	65	Lentils	29	White rice	72
Pineapple	66	Soya beans	15	Brown rice	66
Grapefruit	25			White spaghetti	50
Grapes	46	**Vegetables**		Wholemeal spaghetti	42
		Carrots	49	Cornflakes	80
Sugars		Potatoes (baked)	85	Muesli	66
Glucose	100	Potatoes (fried)	75		
Honey	87	Potatoes (boiled)	70		
Sugar (sucrose)	60	Peas	51		

Water

Water is the ultimate detoxifier! Your thirst mechanism is the body's way of urging you to drink. However, many of us ignore this plea for water, drinking sodas, or tea and coffee instead. By continually failing to heed these thirst signals, the brain will stop sending them out. Instead the body will find other ways of 'borrowing' water from different parts of the body. It will borrow from the skin, hair or wherever else it needs to. When we notice our skin and hair looking dry and drab, we rush out and buy expensive face creams. The best face cream is in your own home in an abundant supply.

Not drinking enough water puts the kidneys under severe pressure as they are not receiving enough water to clear out wastes as efficiently as they should. The best indicator of how your kidneys are working is the colour of your urine. If you are drinking enough water, it should be clear. Dehydration causes constipation and headaches. The little water you do drink will immediately be used to rehydrate your body leaving your kidneys in short supply. Aim to drink at least two litres per day to truly hydrate your body. Once you are in the habit your thirst mechanisms will kick in permanently, making it easier to maintain.

Drinking enough water and taking essential fatty acids will dramatically improve dry skin and hair.

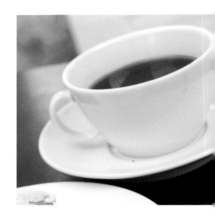

Water retention is a common problem for women especially just before a period. Your weight can go up by as much as five pounds with hands and feet normally swelling. Many women make the mistake of limiting the amount of water they drink in the hope of getting rid of the water retention. However, by doing this, the body assumes a shortage and will hold on to any water, hence the shortage in the first place. Drink more water to flush your system out and reduce your salt intake.

Coffee and tea

It has been branded 'weed killer' by some health experts! Coffee is an addictive drug with no nutritional value. It promotes a stimulating effect of alertness, which is normally followed by a down effect of tiredness encouraging the drinker to have another cup and so the cycle continues. Caffeine also has a diuretic effect on the

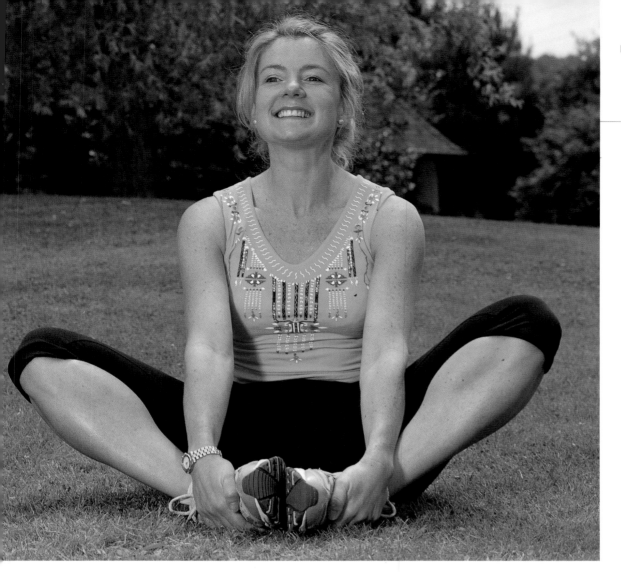

body, which can leave you dehydrated as well as flush vital nutrients out of the body. Tea also contains both caffeine and tannin so, drinking too much will promote the same symptoms as too much coffee. The symptoms that result from too much caffeine are related to heart disease, digestive problems, chronic fatigue, stress, depression, panic attacks, allergies and headaches.

Alcohol

Alcohol contributes to blood-sugar imbalances and excessive drinking can also cause liver damage, weight gain and it is a depressant. My recommendation would be to try and abstain from Monday to Friday and then have a few glasses of wine at the weekend. If you really long for that glass after work every day, make sure that's all it is – a glass. A good way to slow down is to drink a glass of fizzy water between your glasses of wine.

TROUBLESHOOTING

Your questions answered

How should I feel the day after exercising?

Research shows that to have unbearable pain the day after training is not a good thing. This build up of lactic acid, which causes the muscle soreness, inhibits the body from metabolising fat as efficiently as it normally would and, therefore, shuts off fat-burning mechanisms, defeating the object of training in the first place. However, it is not surprising to have some soreness when you first start training as the muscles have been out of action for some time. Once a regular routine is established the muscles will adapt and the soreness will decrease. Your muscles should be comfortably sore the day or two following exercise, just enough that every now and again you can feel you have exercised them.

Can I really change my body shape?

Yes! By being persistent and exercising frequently you will change your body. Many women get impatient and give up on exercise too soon. Provided you are working with correct technique and following the guidelines set out in this book you will start to see changes in your body after just three weeks. After that it just gets better. It is important to combine exercise with proper eating and make lifestyle changes.

Is it better to do cardio or strength training to lose weight?

Both. Cardiovascular burns calories, whilst strength training builds lean tissue revving up the metabolism. A higher metabolic rate burns more calories at rest.

I am exercising but my body is still the same.

Consider the following factors:

• Technique: Are you performing every exercise properly?
• Variety: Are you including cardiovascular and strength training into your programme? Try to do fat-burning exercise for 30–45 minutes, three to five times a week, and some form of strength training at least twice a week.
• Progression: Have you been stuck on the same routine for too long? Try to boost your workout by doing different exercises, using slightly heavier weights or going for more reps.
• Metabolism: Are you eating enough calories to sustain your weekly workouts? Do not under-eat and over-train.
• Types of food: Are you sticking to a sensible diet packed with metabolism-boosting carbohydrates and proteins or are you eating foods with too much fat and sugar?

Is running dangerous for women?

I would not advocate running unless you have strong abdominals, know how to hold yourself properly and are fairly fit. If you possess all of these it is a great way to burn extra calories. It is not advisable to use running as your only form of exercise and many injuries have been caused to runners who do not include strength and flexibility in their training. Make sure you wear proper running shoes, and include a warm up and stretch.

Will I see better results if I join a gym?

The only advantage a gym has is that there is more equipment available, along with classes. You get out of exercise what you put into it. If you find it difficult to motivate yourself then it might be better to join a gym with a friend to keep one another inspired. With a good pair of running/walking shoes, a skipping rope, a set of dumbbells and an exercise ball you have the perfect gym at home. Unless you know how to exercise correctly, the results will be fruitless in a gym or at home.

My knees hurt and prevent me from exercising.

Recent research indicates that both overuse and inactivity can weaken the knee. Inactivity is actually worse because the muscles surrounding the joint become weak and the connective tissue becomes stiff – all of which reduce knee support and range of motion. To avoid injury follow these guidelines:

- Always warm up adequately.
- Strengthen the muscles around the knee including quad, hamstring, inner and outer thigh.
- Vary your activities.
- Invest in good training shoes.
- Ensure proper technique, especially when doing lunges and squats.

My back hurts.

Back pain will almost surely become a thing of the past if you strengthen your abdominal muscles by working them correctly on a regular basis and stretching other muscles. In addition, tight hamstrings and hip flexors are attributed to back pain. Sitting all day long tends to tighten up the hip flexors in particular. It is vital to stretch both them and the hamstring muscles frequently.

How do I get rid of my stomach?

Make sure you are exercising aerobically three to five times a week to burn body fat. When you do exercise your stomach muscles ensure you are working all four muscle groups correctly, keeping those abdominals zipped up all the time. Make sure your diet is not too high in fat or sugar.

Common weight-related ailments

Digestive problems and bloating

Digestive problems and bloating can be caused by stress. Eating when you are stressed is not advisable mainly because the adrenal glands are put under severe demands causing a less efficient digestive system. Food particles go undigested causing bloating, stomach aches, back or shoulder pain, headaches and even allergies. Another cause of digestive problems is eating on the run. If you do not have the time to sit down and eat slowly don't eat at all. Try to chew each mouthful about ten times before swallowing – this goes a long way to helping the digestive system work optimally.

Chewing gum

Chewing gum on an empty stomach could cause bloating. If you are going to chew gum, then only chew it after a meal. When you chew gum on an empty stomach the digestive juices start flowing in the anticipation of a meal to follow. Valuable digestive enzymes go wasted and then when a meal is taken in, their capacity is depleted. If my clients suffer from bloating or stress I have suggested that they take digestive enzymes at the onset of a meal. They have all reported an immense improvement.

Premenstrual syndrome

Premenstrual syndrome is characterised by a number of distressing symptoms prior to menstruation. These symptoms can be physically related such as fluid retention, breast tenderness, bloating and food (particularly sugar) cravings, or emotionally charged such as depression, anxiety and irritability. Many women are plagued every month for up to two weeks, which makes life difficult to get on with, especially if you are trying to keep in shape.

If you suffer from irritability, nausea, headaches or migraines before your period it can often be traced to a congested liver. A traditional herbal remedy that works well on the liver is milk thistle. If you suffer from painful breasts, mood swings and most of the symptoms associated with PMS the best herbal remedy I know of is *Agnus castus*. This powerful herb really works! Vitamin B6 and essential fatty acids are important for treating PMS.

Anaemia

This is quite common amongst women, particularly those who have had a few children. Typical symptoms are exhaustion and feeling dizzy. Even if you are eating an iron-rich diet, chances are that your body is losing more iron than it should. This could be through heavy periods, or exercise. Tea and coffee also deplete the body's iron stores. If you think you are suffering from anaemia go and have a blood test. If you are, take a non-constipating iron supplement or extra Vitamin C with iron.

Headaches

It always surprises me when people assume one headache a week is the norm. If you get more than four headaches a year, there is an underlying cause. Stress can cause tension headaches but the most common cause is normally dehydration.

Depression

If depression is affecting your weight by sending you straight to the fridge, and you are finding it difficult to break this vicious cycle, then it is worth taking some positive action – naturally. The herb St John's wort (Hypericum) has had a superb success rate in relieving mild or moderately severe depression with no side effects. It is also most helpful in relieving the symptoms of seasonal affective disorder (SAD). Exercise has been shown to greatly improve the symptoms of depression and even though it is the last thing you feel like doing, making the effort will elevate your mood considerably. I also find aromatherapy oils such as rosemary and bergamot help to lift your mood.

Constipation

If you do not open your bowels at least once, preferably twice, a day then you are constipated. The major causes of constipation are going on fad diets – the body simply has no idea when the next meal will be and bowels become sluggish – and not drinking enough water. Increasing your intake of fresh fruit and vegetables and taking one tablespoon of linseeds in your cereal or yogurt is helpful.

DON'T LOOK BACK

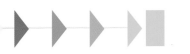

By now you should be fully aware that we are not going to venture down the quick diet or exercise route. Although this may not be what you want to hear initially, I am convinced that once you understand my formula for success and implement it into your lifestyle you will never look back. Remember this is not quick fix system – it's a forever fix system.

It's time to stop feeling bad about yourself. It's time to stop being tired of being tired. It's time to start the healing process. For the first time in your life you are going to combine sensible eating with exercise and stick with it. As you begin to feel better with increased energy levels it will motivate you to carry on.

Save yourself from years of misery by following the Jenergy principles

- Technique – focus your mind and position your body correctly.
- Strength training – the only long-term fat buster.
- A woman only approach to a better body – fit, firm and feminine.
- Maximise your fat blast with cardiovascular exercise – walking, running, cycling, skipping and rollerblading.
- DIET: Don't . . . It Ends In Tears – increase your metabolic rate and burn more calories at rest.

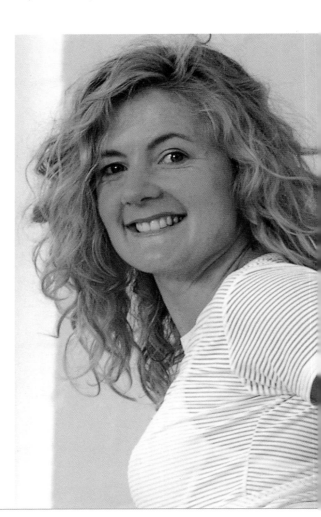

Progression training

Once you achieve your fitness goals you can either maintain them by keeping your fitness at its current level or change your existing exercise routine. If you are feeling bored, unmotivated or just not seeing the desired results then it's time to change your resistance and cardiovascular training programme. Cross training is an excellent way to challenge your body to new levels and prevent boredom as well as being time efficient. By placing new challenges on your body you will improve and the fitter you get the easier it becomes. Douglas Brooks promotes variety as the name of the game for optimal muscular development. 'It seems that the best stimulus for increasing strength gains is to make the muscles work harder, as opposed to longer,' he says.

The outdoor workouts in this book are challenging. Once you understand the key to fitness you can devise your own workouts. If your chosen activity is always walking then introduce short bursts of running to improve your aerobic capacity. Add stairs, skipping, swimming or rollerblading and push your body just that little bit further. It is important to vary your routines. Cross training and interval training are both great.

Increase your weight or the amount of reps you perform. A good indicator of improving your strength gains is to take the muscles out of their comfort zone. Just when you think you cannot do another rep, do an additional four.

A realistic approach

A sure sign that you're going to fail is to use the 'diet' word. A recent study on people and how they diet showed that an overwhelming majority of people who start on diets give up within a few months. Another study tracked down people with successful weight loss and asked them what they did. It certainly wasn't the cabbage diet or slimming pills. Those people who had successfully kept their weight off for five years or more all did the same thing. They changed their eating habits for life and started exercising regularly. It's your choice. Either carry on with your stop-start regime forever or move onto a realistic approach and throw those scales away.

This realistic approach to a better relationship with your body is attainable to women of all ages. Find out what works for you and start right now, with every intention of achieving what you've never been able to in the past.

Acknowledgements

I would like to take this opportunity to thank
everyone who has been instrumental in putting this
book together.

To Lorraine Kelly, Wilma Kaufmann, Mags Levin, and
Sarka Kartakova for being such fine examples of what the
Jenergy programme can do for you. To Guy Hearn for his
amazingly creative photography and thanks to Richard
Sinclair for the use of his beautiful studio. To Fit Kit for
supplying the clothing.

I'd like to thank my literary agents Araminta Whitley and Celia
Hayley at Lucas Alexander Whitley for believing in my work and
wanting to promote my unique programme to women nationwide.

To everyone at HarperCollins*Publishers* who have been fantastic
to work with and I'd like to thank them all, especially Victoria
Alers-Hankey for all her hard effort and enthusiasm.

Without the experience of having worked with many women
who have switched to my programme, Jenergy would not
have been possible, so thanks to all my devotees. To my
friends and family who have been enormously supportive
– especially by beautiful daughter Kirsti.

Ultimately, I give thanks to God for the inner
strength, peace and wisdom he has taught me.